CW00602919

I'd Love To, But What'll I Wear?

I'd Love To, But What'll I Wear?

POLLY BERGEN

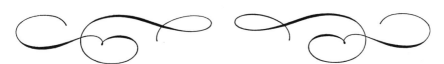

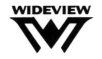

WIDEVIEW

"After the Christening" on page 73, copyright 1934 by Ogden Nash. From *The Face Is Familiar* by Ogden Nash, by permission of Little, Brown and Co.

Copyright © 1977 by Polly Bergen and Kathrin Perutz.

All rights reserved. No part of this book may be reproduced, stored in a retrieval system or transmitted in any form by an electronic, mechanical, photocopying, recording means or otherwise, without prior written permission of the author. For information contact Wyden Books, 747 Third Avenue, New York, N.Y. 10017. Printed in the United States of America.

First Wyden Books edition: June 1977

First Wideview edition: October 1978

Library of Congress Cataloging in Publication Data

Bergen, Polly, 1930–
  I'd love to, but what'll I wear?

      1. Fashion.   2. Clothing and dress.   I. Perutz, Kathrin, 1939–   joint author.   II. Title.
  TT507.B44   646'.34   77–2125
  ISBN: 0–87223–523–8

Contents

Contents

Contents

I'd Love To, But What'll I Wear?

Introduction

Ever since Eve plucked the apple in Eden and cried, "I haven't a thing to wear!", women have echoed her. Through the ages, since Paradise, women have made their lament to half-empty closets and crowded dressing rooms; to husbands, lovers and friends; to salespeople, mothers of the bride, tour directors and, mainly, to themselves. It's said daily by rich women, poor women, old ones, young ones and women who claim no age.

It's never literally true (except possibly in the case of Eve), but is always sincere. It can mean many things: "I'm bored with all the clothes I have and this is an opportunity to buy something new." Or: "He's already seen me in everything I want him to see me in." Or: "With my weight gain/loss nothing fits properly anymore." Or: "I feel like a new person today and I don't want to wear hand-me-downs from the person I used to be."

Whatever the cause, it's always a cry for help: TELL ME WHAT TO WEAR! And yet—as many women know and some men discover —the only acceptable answer is one that finds an echo in the woman herself; she is asking to be told something she already suspects to be right.

Introduction

Today it's harder to go by the rule than at any other time in history, since the rules of dressing have been relaxed to a point where you often can't tell what they are at all. Even the restaurant signs requiring jackets, ties or "appropriate dress" are disappearing, and the world of fashion has become a wonderful, colorful, devil-may-care bonanza which seems to offer total liberation. That makes it even more difficult to know what's right. With all the choices, possibilities and varieties in clothes, it's hard to figure out the *unstated* rules. A woman is left on her own, without guidelines.

Although the world of clothing and fashion has become very relaxed and given us freedom to express ourselves, it's not always easy to say what you mean. Clothes are a statement you make about who you are—about who you'd like people to think you are. Unless you can make that statement in a straightforward way, people are likely to get the wrong message.

Your appearance projects your personality and your individuality. It takes years of living and experience to develop a style in any art, and if it's the art of dressing, don't expect to develop an individual style overnight. It took me a long time, even though I had been in the public eye for many years before that, and was receiving advice from knowledgeable people. I started in show business at the age of fifteen. I sang with bands, made movies, appeared in nightclubs and on television. I dressed for public appearances almost every day, but didn't develop a style of dressing that made a statement about who I was until nearly two decades later.

Before that, I made a lot of mistakes. Mistakes in dressing happen when you're trying for an appearance that is basically not who you are. When I was very young, first starting in show business, my greatest wish was to be Hedy Lamarr or Lana Turner. It was very important to me to be sexy and slinky and sophisticated. And, because my knowledge of what was sexy, slinky and sophisticated came only from films I'd seen, I tried to imitate that image.

Introduction

At the age of fifteen, I made my first really important purshase. It was a dress of black crepe, slinky and draped, with a very, very low V-neck, tiny straps over the shoulders, a very bare back, and absolutely form-fitting all the way down. I wore long rhinestone earrings, and carried a cigarette holder with a cigarette in it. That was my way of looking as I wanted to look. It was glamorous. It also solved a basic problem I had, working in places where I was underage. This made me look older. There I was, a chubby, baby-fat fifteen-year-old girl walking into a nightclub to be interviewed as a band singer in slinky black crepe with long rhinestone earrings and my hair all swept to one side over one ear. I wonder what people thought.

But to me this was the way Hedy Lamarr looked. As a matter of fact, I think I got the outfit after seeing her in *White Cargo*. And it worked—the job was mine.

I always had a tendency to overdress. I didn't understand simple understated chic—I didn't even know what that meant. In my early and mid twenties I began to learn more and more about dressing, but my tendency was to rely on what other people told me and not to trust my own instincts. Not until my thirties did I start to achieve a look for myself that I felt comfortable with. And remember, I was exposed to the great fashion designers of major studios—in particular Edith Head, who designed everything from cowgirl outfits to royal robes—years before that. No wonder I finally learned how.

It has always been important for me to know how to dress. As entertainer or businesswoman, I've been the object of careful scrutiny. On stage, on television or at a board meeting, I've had to project an image of who I am. The fact that I'm now secure about my own style says a lot about the way I feel within myself. As a young woman in the movies, I tried to fit into a mold. My style of dressing was a type of costume, to conform with a preconceived image. Now that I'm older and more independent, the way I dress is a projection of how I see myself, and how I want others to see me.

Introduction

Before you can be concerned with individual style, you have to have
a sense of what to wear when. Women are sometimes embarrassed because they don't know what to put on. They feel ridiculous or insecure
or stupid because they can't settle on exactly the right thing at the
right time. There's no need to feel that. All you need is a little encouragement in the direction of your own instincts.

Don't be intimidated by fashion, or by other women who are good
dressers, or by magazine articles, or by men and their attitudes toward
dressing. You know yourself, and it's my hope that this book will give
you the confidence and assurance you need to make a fashion statement
that's right for you—regardless of what is considered the "in" thing.

Everyone makes mistakes. The awful thing about a mistake is that
you find out only after it's been made, after that terrible moment when
you know you're all wrong. I could tell a hundred stories about my
mistakes, but another woman is not going to learn too much from
hearing about them, because they're not *her* mistakes. The point is that
everyone makes them, and there's no need to feel insecure because you
don't instantly know what is the "right" thing to wear.

We're given a lot of freedom in dressing nowadays, and we can use
it to our advantage. We can indulge in fantasies, change our moods,
conceal our defects and say who we are. With just a litle guidance about
unspoken rules (no exposed navel at a wedding, for instance), you
should be able to set your mind at rest and start building up a wardrobe
of clothes that you're comfortable with and feel right about. You'll be
making your statement, and the message will come across: Here I am.
This is *me*. People will probably think that's pretty terrific.

I

The Joy of Clothing

Each of us is a lot of different selves. We're all multifaceted, and behind every "you" there's another "you" waiting to come out. We have different moods, in the course of a life or in the course of a day, depending on whom we're with, what we're doing, where we are. Clothes let us say different things about ourselves at different times.

What you wear is the first statement you make to people you meet. Just because it's a first, it's a very strong statement indeed, and it gives away a lot about you. That's why dressing is an art: You're telling the world something about yourself. You're expressing yourself in a nonverbal way, and you have to decide what your message is.

I can walk into a restaurant at midday and tell you which women are having business lunches, and which women are there for pleasure. Their way of dressing gives them away.

Everybody reacts to that. If you see a woman in a vampish outfit, you'll make very specific judgments about her as a woman. You may not be completely right—maybe she's just play-acting—but your judgments are correct insofar as this is how she is presenting herself right then. You probably wouldn't trust her as your banker, you wouldn't

7

want to invite her to a Mother's Day celebration, and you'd be definitely uneasy if she was your child's schoolteacher.

Clothing might be a necessity in cold climates, but we hardly ever wear clothes just for warmth. Dressing is an elaborate game that all humans learn to play. It's the oldest of all games, played wherever people live. The rules change with time, place and life-style, but the object is always to say something about yourself. Fashion as a whole is revealing of the time we live in and the general way of life. Individual dressing and style will show your status, your personal life-style, your background perhaps, your expectations, where you came from, what you do.

What you say about yourself can be true or false, but you should make a conscious choice and not let it be misleading. You can learn to play your own look against the general fashion background, with small adaptations to the area or country you're in.

How you dress will depend basically on emotional, psychological and financial factors—how you feel about yourself, what impression you want to make, how much you can afford to spend on clothes. Your budget will make a difference, of course, in what clothes you buy, but the difference will probably be more in fabrics than styles.

You must feel comfortable about your clothes and in your clothes. You should think about clothes up to the time you put them on, and then forget about them. They should let you be free to be yourself—or whatever self you have chosen to be at that time. Once it was that clothes made the man and women made the clothes. Now, clothes reflect the person.

I used to buy only "showstoppers"—outfits that knocked you out when I walked into a room. Now, I don't want to wear anything that enters a room ahead of me. I don't want an outfit that makes its own announcement. I'd prefer wearing something that's part of me, Polly, and allows me to come through as a person.

Some of my friends are what I call "serious" dressers, and they almost invariably dress wrong. I mean those people who want the security of an outfit, who'll buy something because they've seen it in a magazine, or because it has the "right" label. This shows a lack of personal identity. They're saying that they have no real sense of themselves. They'll wear a Galanos dress which might look terrible on them, but they're secure because the label says Galanos. Some of the Beautiful People belong in this category—they let the dress wear them instead of the other way around.

I love clothes. I love the fun of dressing, of being able to express myself and the different parts of my personality. I like dressing in the morning for work, and then later in the day adding jewelry or accessories, removing something, moving something else around for a softer look. Dressing should be fun and creative. In the art of dressing, as in any other art, personal style is what counts.

What You Wear Is Who You Are

Even your innermost feelings about yourself come through in your clothes and the way you carry them. Whenever I enter a room, I hold myself as tall as I can. I want people to notice that I'm here, so even if I'll be slouching through the rest of the meeting or lunch, I enter like a queen, and I give a first impression of confidence and self-assurance.

People react to that immediately. They pay closer attention to you, they listen harder, they're quicker in offering services. When you and your clothes are giving a picture of importance, you're treated as though you are important.

But even if you're on stilts, you won't counteract the effect of a slinky sheath bared to the belly or sloppy jeans with patches interspersed between the rips. You want to develop your own style, but if it's completely eccentric, you have to be able to carry it off or not care what anyone thinks.

Aim for an appearance that says who you are and makes the most of it. You'll discover that certain clothes are right for you. Try a lot of them, in different colors and styles, until you find those that always seem to look the best on you, from your point of view. You'll find that these are usually the things you're most comfortable in as well. And probably these clothes will earn you the most compliments. Take notice of the compliments you get, and for which outfits. You'll see that the compliments are consistent for a look that is yours, that works for you.

It works if it accords with your own self-image. That may be slightly idealized, and it will be—should be—evolving, in the way that you evolve. You may be basically the same person at forty that you were at twenty, but many facets will have deepened, many priorities will have changed. Your outside appearance evolves along with your inner development.

And, because you're never exactly the same person in all situations, your look will change depending on where you are and the mood you're in. "Who do I want to be for this occasion?" you ask yourself. Should I come across as a no-nonsense businesswoman? A concerned parent? An adorable or provocative woman? A responsible citizen? A good sport? You make that decision first, and dress accordingly. How successful you've been in conveying that image will be apparent partly in the way people react to you and partly in the way you feel about yourself.

Aspects of your personality change with time and according to the occasion. Your mood may be different at lunch than at dinner. But underneath these changes, you are still you, an individual, and no one else is exactly like you. The same is true for outward appearance. Your look alters with the event, but your style is your own, and style—like personality—is the product of living, of countless experiences, mistakes and decisions. It's what you're telling others about yourself.

The Joy of Clothing

When my oldest daughter, Kathy, visited me recently, she said something that made me realize my statement was coming across: "Mom, you've really developed a way to look that is yours. It's your style."

A style that is yours. It'll be the way you look nine times out of ten no matter what you put on, from the most elaborate evening gown to the simplest pants and top. You might not notice it yourself even, but others will. I've just recognized that for the past ten or more years I consistently wear one style more than any other. I hadn't thought it out for myself—I wasn't conscious of selecting a particular style—but because I pretty much know what will work for me and what won't, I tend to get the same type of thing every time I shop.

The other day I went into a store to try on evening dresses. The first was a very stuffy gown. The second was a simple, high-necked, long-sleeved red chiffon dress cut on the bias, with a red chiffon stole to match. I had it on, and it looked so much like so many things I own (except that I have nothing in fire engine red) that I just felt yes, well it's kinda nice, but . . .

So I went on with the clothes, trying on at least a dozen and ending up ultimately with something devastating I'd seen on a model in *Vogue.* I was about to get it, but somehow or other I knew that, devastating as the gown was—and it was—the combination of it and me was not the best. Good, but not tops.

So I went back to the second dress I had on, which was similar to so many things I had hanging in my closet. I recognized that it was me. I bought that red dress, I've worn it and I know I'll wear it and wear it until I wear it out. The other dress I would have worn maybe once a year, and it would have made a strong fashion statement. It was obviously "designed." It had a very specific designer's look to it. Maybe that's what turned me off at the end—*the statement it was making belonged to the designer and not to me.*

How do you know what's *you* in clothes? You read through the magazines, look at lots of pictures, go window-shopping and see what other women are wearing. But most important, you have to physically put the clothes on your body. That's the only way you'll know what best reflects you and the way you feel about yourself.

Don't be too conservative. I've never stopped experimenting with clothes, and you won't either. Fashion is always offering something new, or something revived. Try out the latest colors in accessories—you can create new looks each year for the same basic outfits by fashionable touches here and there. Fashion changes all the time, as you yourself are changing. You go through new and different experiences that influence you as a person, your outlook and your view of clothes. Though you remain with the same basic style, you'll always be making new adaptations, new changes.

Look at a few standard items of wear, like jeans or a business suit. Millions of people dress in the same basic garment, but they can still have an individual look. Even the exact same pair of jeans can express different personalities, depending on who wears them. Jeans say, I'm young; or, I want you to think I'm young; or, I feel young. Jeans also express casualness, naturalness, comfort and conformity. Most young people wear jeans, and no wonder. Young people, who are not often sure which of their many selves is the real one, tend to conform in dress to help them gain the assurance that they belong, and to tell outsiders that they're part of a group.

Beyond that, they do want to express themselves. Which is why they make serious choices about minute aspects of the jeans: what color and material; where the waist should be, how the legs should be cut. Then they add embroidery, patches, studs or rhinestones. They write their names or a message in thread, paint or metal. They let the pants get very old, or they press them. Each of these variations is an expression of individuality.

If we see two identical pairs of jeans—faded blue, fly zipper, waist at the waistline, stove-pipe legs—we will react to them differently if one pair is on a sixteen-year-old girl, the other on a sixty-year-old woman. The older woman is making a very definite statement, and our reaction will depend on how appropriate we feel it is. If we meet her in jeans on a walk through the woods, we get a different impression than if we meet her in the same outfit at an elegant luncheon. In the first instance her statement is, "I'm here for exercise, I'm wearing the most comfortable thing I own, and I'm not trying to give out a fashion message." In the second instance, she's obviously not dressed appropriately, and is making a strong statement about her feeling of losing her youth. She's showing contempt for her surroundings (maybe also for her lunch partner) by wearing a garment not intended for this situation. She's drawing attention to herself, and it's mostly negative.

The equivalent to jeans in the woods is a well-cut suit or simple dress in the restaurant. If she wore a navy knit suit at lunch, she wouldn't be the center of attention, but she could be making a fashion statement through the blouse, scarf, shoes, bag, jewelry or whatever accessories she had selected to create a total look.

If you wear a bright red top to work, you want others to think you're happy. Red is a signal for a mood. But what you wear that top with, and how you wear it will be making an even stronger statement. Just as each person has a distinctive way of speaking, so each person has, or can have, a distinctive way of using the language of clothes.

Building a Wardrobe

For some women, each deterioration in a marriage brings an improvement in their wardrobe. When you're down, clothes can give you a lift. You buy them because you're depressed and you want to change your mood, get something new, pick yourself up and start all over again.

If you have a large clothes budget, this can be a simple and effective way to cheer yourself up. But if you can't afford to buy clothes you might not need, try to restrain yourself. You're looking for something new and different to help bring you out of yourself, and it may not be the best for you. You'll have a tendency to shop with reduced judgment, without considering whether a spur-of-the-moment purchase will go with other things you have, and you may never wear it again.

When your lover has gone or the job you were waiting for doesn't come off, treat yourself to a shopping spree only if you have the money to buy whatever appeals to you on the spot, knowing that a lot of it will never be worn, will be thrown out, or will have to be exchanged. I know. It's happened to me. I buy when I'm depressed and then later I'm depressed by what I bought. It's best to treat yourself to only a few fantasy or luxury items.

To get the most for your money, and have the most effective wardrobe you can afford, start by making a list. Go through everything you have and see what that gives you. Coordinate as you itemize. What about the shocking pink blouse that won't go with anything? If you love it, you'll need a skirt or pants to wear with it. Otherwise, give it away. Many women say they have "nothing to wear" just because their clothes don't match. They may have eighteen skirts—but only one they ever put on.

Remove all those things you know you're not going to wear—ever. I know this is one of the hardest jobs in the world, but try. Something you bought ten years ago and have only worn twice still looks new and great. But ask yourself why you haven't worn it. If the answer is that it's out of style and looks hopelessly dated, think of ways you could adapt it. I was throwing out all my minis when the miniskirt fashion had passed, until I realized those little dresses could work as tunics over skirts or pants. Some had to be shortened slightly.

If you can adapt a garment so it's acceptable for present fashion, do it. Don't wait until the great wheel of fashion revolves around again to that particular style. Sometimes it happens in a few years; sometimes it takes decades, occasionally centuries; and once in a while it's a flash in the pan that never recurs. But also, since fashion is so very permissive now, there are many clothes you can take out of the attic and wear to a party. Or your daughter, sister, friend or mother can use them. Many women adore antique clothes, and they're fun for an evening out, or in.

Try wearing something you don't use anymore for a different purpose than was originally intended. Take that beautiful old silk blouse with ruffles. It looks overdressed with any skirt you have, but it might be perfect with jeans, which will balance it out.

That ten-year-old thing is still hanging there, and you're still undecided. The color is so fabulous and unusual—you've never seen anything else in that shade of purple. Maybe that's the problem. The color doesn't work on you. It overpowers you, or does something funny to your skin tone. In that case, get rid of it, no matter how perfect its condition. Get rid of it also if it doesn't fit properly and never has. Maybe you bought it impetuously, or were given it as a present. It never looked right on you. Out it goes, even if you're determined to lose twenty pounds or take up body-building. You and it are incompatible, and there's no point cluttering the closet.

All right, now you've been very strong and thrown out everything you haven't worn in five years. The closet looks emptier, and you feel justice has been on your side all along when you said you needed new clothes and your husband said your closets were jammed so you wouldn't even have room for anything new. There's room now. But here comes the most difficult of all tasks: throwing out your favorites. That baby-blue sweater dress brings out your eyes. Whenever you wear it you receive compliments and you know you're looking as good as you possibly can. That dress brought you three new lovers, and you rely on it when you want to make a new conquest.

Only trouble is, the dress has had it. It's worn out, and the shape is gone. You know it has to go, but you can't bear it. It's like parting with your closest friend, one who makes you feel and look your best.

Take the dress to your "little dressmaker" or tailor and have it copied. Then have copies made in other colors and materials. That's what I do with my all-time favorites if I can't replace them with anything in the stores. But I won't wear anything that's beat-up, no matter how much I once loved it.

Most women, I think, are superstitious about clothes. Certain garments seem to have a kind of magic to them. They look sensational, and always work. This can be a dress, a top, even underwear. They're special clothes that do special things, and sometimes you feel you can't risk their magic by wearing them for commonplace events. You won't wear those satin underpants to work, even if they're the only clean pair you've got. They're too powerful, somehow—they've only been worn on certain occasions, when you hoped they would be seen, and they always were. That shimmering top was worn to a reception where you met Him, and the next time you had it on, it landed you the job you have now.

Almost everyone has such clothes, with some kind of magic to them, and we hang on to them long after its possible to wear them. Then we have the reverse kind of clothes: things that look perfectly all right on the hanger—of a good material, fashionable, in perfect condition—and yet they never work. Whenever you wear such an outfit, something unpleasant occurs. The evening turns out to be a bore, the play you're seeing is horrible, the food you ordered arrives cold, or the man you're with cools off.

I have an outfit that's accident-prone. Whenever I wear it, something happens—wine spills on it, food plops on it. I'm never in it for long before the accident occurs. I'm not accident-prone, but the outfit is, and it needs dry cleaning after every wear. I can't explain it and what's worse, I love the dumb thing.

The Joy of Clothing

You should go through your closet a minimum of once every six months—if possible every three or four months—and weed out whatever's of no use. The easiest time to do this, I've found, is when you're moving. In fact, that's the only time I really complete the job. Of course, this requires a lot of moving and may not be practical for you.

OK, let's say now you've done it. You have only clothes you can and do wear, with perhaps your wedding dress in the attic, or a ball gown for that once-in-ten-years possibility. Now make your list, showing each type of garment you own, and how many of each. How many more of that kind do you require? Are three skirts enough? Are they all everyday skirts? Then you need something dressier for evening.

What will go with what? Do you have bags and shoes to go with every outfit? How about the little things—hose, underpants, bras. Do you have an adequate supply? Are you bored with any of your outfits? Do they need a lift? A new scarf might do the trick, or a brightly colored belt, or a new blouse to wear with the suit that looks fine with the mustard-colored top you always wear with it (but the problem is you *always* wear that top).

You're ready to shop. You know what you have, and how many items in each category. You also know how much you can afford to spend. If it's not enough to get everything you need all at once, star the items that are most essential. The amount of money you have to spend on clothes will naturally make the biggest difference in the size of the investment you make. If you're a woman with a really large clothes allowance—as I have had in my life; as a Jacqueline Onassis has—then you can afford to buy the showstoppers, because you can buy a different showstopper for every occasion when you walk into a room full of people.

But if you can't afford it, stick to basics. With a little imagination, you can dress up most outfits and change them around. The women I know who have really great style rarely change their way of dressing.

It's very consistent over the years and almost looks as though they always have the same thing on—except they don't. There's always some nuance that makes it fresh and new.

Once you know what you need and what you can afford, think of your body, your life-style and your personality—or the one you want to project. If you're overweight, forget about little box jackets; if your life-style is very active, don't buy clothes so extremely tailored that they'll constrict you. Hopefully, the personality you wish to project will be a part of who you are. If you're a basically conservative woman wearing a very bare, provocative dress, you'll be presenting a picture of yourself so far from who you really are that it can get you in a lot of trouble. (This is okay, if you're looking for trouble.)

So be aware of your clothing needs, your financial limits, how you live, who you are and how you're built. The essential wardrobe will differ from one person to another depending on many additional factors, such as the climate you live in, the kind of work you do and the sort of social life you have.

Try never to buy emotionally and, if possible, never at the last minute. If you're buying under pressure, you may end up with something that's just right for one particular occasion, but will never be worn again. Or you choose something you saw in a magazine because you're desperate for *something*, even though you don't really have time to consider whether or not it's right for you.

Shop in advance of the season, if possible. Go by a specific list of your requirements for that season. If you need a winter coat, don't drift through the beach-wear section (you might fall in love with something!).

Before going on a trip, decide whether you want to make shopping a part of your vacation. Unlike most women I know, I almost never shop in Europe. I hate shopping, so I'll buy my French sportswear and my Italian bathing suits before I leave for France or Italy. I feel that if I'm going for a vacation, the one thing that will spoil it is shopping. So while other women are rummaging in stores, trying to get someone to wait on them in the midst of the tourist season, I'm lying in the sun on the sand with a cool drink in my hand, having a wonderful time.

I realize this makes me different from most people. If you love to shop, do make it part of your trip. Don't buy the trench coat here— wait for London. If you plan to buy clothes from European designers, wait till you're in their boutiques. You'll have more fun, and something special to look forward to. Don't plan to shop abroad, though, as an economy move. Some things may be less expensive there, but others will cost the same or even more. Sometimes clothes designed for export are commissioned, mass-produced and therefore less expensive in the country to which they're shipped than in the country where they're made. This doesn't go for native dress, of course, and if you love Moroccan tunics, wait till you're in Tangiers or Marrakesh to buy them. You'll find a larger selection and will be able to buy half a dozen for the price of two at home.

Even if you're traveling in this country, you can save some of your shopping till you get where you're going. If you live far from a city, then shopping in large department stores may be an exciting change. Perhaps you'll want to go to Neiman-Marcus in Dallas, and you'll want a project when you get there. Hold off on the belt, or bag, or extra top, and treat yourself to a morning of browsing with a specific purchase in mind.

I don't recommend, however, that you travel without essentials. Even if you plan to do all your shopping in New York, or Paris, or Los Angeles, take along at least the barest minimum of necessary clothes so you won't be forced into impetuous buying because you really have nothing along that will take you through an evening.

As I said before, essentials will vary with each woman. But every woman, no matter who or where, needs the following rock-bottom inventory (unless she's planning to live like Robinson Crusoe):

Undergarments. Bras, panties, hose.

Nightclothes. Gowns or pj's and a pretty robe that will go with all of them and look at least presentable if you receive an unexpected visitor. Loose, long robes, caftans or kimonos are best. After all, you can't receive room service in the nude.

Day Wear

Day bag. A roomy handbag, preferably black or tan, to go with everything.

Shoes. Two pairs—one black, the other camel-colored, well-fitting and with a comfortable heel.

Dress. Shirtwaist, sweater dress or other simple cut for work or lunch, in a color that suits you. The simpler the dress, the more you'll be able to do with it.

Suit. Get your suit or skirt and jacket in a nonseasonal fabric, like gabardine, light wool or a knit. If you can get a three- or four-piece outfit (skirt, jacket, pants, vest), you can take it a long way.

Skirts and/or pants. Two for daily wear.

Jacket. Two are preferable—one in wool, the other in velvet. If you can only invest in one, make it a light wool that goes with your skirts, pants and dresses.

Shirt/blouse. Man-tailored silk or silk-synthetic shirts are the most versatile, can be dressed up or down. You'll need more tops than bottoms, so if your budget is extremely limited, get a couple of good skirts, with half a dozen tops. Each top should go with each of the two skirts.

Sweaters. Depending on the climate you live in, you'll need anywhere from two to a dozen. But everyone must have at least one cardigan (for cover-up in air conditioning or on cool days), and one other simple sweater, turtleneck or crew neck.

Winter coat. Where applicable.

Evening Wear

Dinner dresses. At least two. This is the simple, fluid dress that will go anywhere from an elegant luncheon to a dinner party.

Long dress. Choose from among all the loose, flowing styles—caftans, long T-shirts, shirtwaists or sweater dresses, if they're not clinging. Depending on your kind of social life, you'll get this dress in a fabric ranging from cotton to satin brocade. If money is tight, make sure you choose a nonseasonal fabric so the dress can take you through the year.

Long skirt. Simple cut or peasant type, to dress up or down depending on the top.

Dressy pants. If you have only one pair to get, make it black velvet. That goes with everything, and is sensational with a silk or satin blouse.

Pajamas. Extremely useful for at-home entertaining, for evening at someone else's home or, if simple enough, a restaurant.

Cocktail dress. Optional. Dressier than the dinner dress, it's often décolleté and quite formal. Not for at-homes.

Evening gown. Optional. You're probably better off buying an extra-long dress or skirt and dressing it up, if necessary, with jewelry.

Evening shoes. Flesh-colored. For a second pair, get gold or silver, or even better, a combination of both.

Evening bag. Gold, silver, black.

Summer Wear

General. Sundress, skirts, shorts, bathing suits, one cover-up, large scarves to wrap around hips, waist or shoulders. Sandals, straw hat. Important item: stole or shawl for summer evenings or air conditioning.

Duster/raincoat. A lightweight, unlined silk coat that doubles as summer coat and raincoat.

In addition, you'll have casual pants or jeans. The preceding list is only a broad outline; just about everyone will need at least one of each of the items, and everyone will need more than one of many of them.

In general, when you're shopping, check out the fabric. Will it flow on you or bind? It's very important to get clothes that don't wrinkle. No matter how beautiful the outfit, it's worthless if every time you sit down you'll get up looking as though you just got out of bed. Always remember, with whatever you're buying: Give that outfit a fast run of your life-style in the dressing room. Take special care with pants and skirts that look heavenly when you're standing up. Sitting down, you might find those pants are too tight in the crotch. Or that divine skirt rides up too far, so you're suddenly wearing a skirt that's halfway up your thighs, even though it came below your knees when you were standing up. If you spend your day at a desk, be extra-careful. You may be making a totally different statement after sitting all day than the one you started out making, and probably wanted to make.

Also: Check the label for care of a garment. If it specifies dry cleaning, you know that this is not something you'll want to take traveling. If you plan to wear it often, the upkeep may end up costing more than the trip.

Consider color—whether it suits you, whether it will go with other things you own, and how easy it is to keep clean. Very light colors might not look crisp at the end of a workday if you're riding subways and taking buses; and you know black can be a problem because it collects lint.

Remember when women believed in "basic black"? Long before the slogan, "Black is beautiful," black was the solution to most dressing problems and was always considered elegant. It certainly is elegant, and beautiful and basic—but so are many other colors that are easier to keep fresh. Black does have a particular quality (which it shares with white). Many women look their best in it, because black (or white) brings out facial coloring. Warm skin tones look marvelous against black. A sleeveless black dress will make the most of your peaches-and-cream tan.

So don't feel that black is out simply because it's no longer the regulation uniform for cocktail parties. The little black dress, the sheer black negligee, the black bra and panties are all sensational—*if* they're for you. If not, you can be just as sexy in sheer red or blue or beige, and the little black dress is equally elegant in beige or burgundy or chocolate brown.

Build up a wardrobe of clothes you'll get the most use out of. Make sure they're comfortable (most important!), easy to care for and chic. If you move in the direction of understatement, you'll have no problem.

Clothes are wonderful. They can give you a lift, change your mood, even create fantasies. Clothes let you be who you want to be, from hausfrau to madam. They're a way of speaking to the world about yourself. If you're not interested in clothes at all, chances are you're not much interested in anything else, either. Since all the world's a stage, we'll get most pleasure out of life by dressing for all the roles we have to play.

Wearing Thin and Other Tricks

Clothes should make the most of what you have, but if what you have is too much, they should make the least of it.

All of us have some problems and some beautiful features. In planning for clothes, we should first take stock of our assets and liabilities, and choose the styles, colors and cuts that make the most of the pluses and minimize the minuses.

The Duchess of Windsor once said that no woman can be too thin or too rich and she has been on the list of the world's ten best-dressed women with the inevitability of Christmas. Thinness may be a problem in other ways, but it's not a fashion problem. If you're thin, most of fashion is perfect for you. The Lord may have taken away, but you've been given magnificent freedom to wear just about anything. And if you do want to add, that's not difficult. It's always possible to pad, but it's not easy to remove.

All the suggestions in this book apply to everyone—all figure types, heights, ages and economic levels. But, just as you might have to buy a less expensive version of an outfit because your budget won't allow rich fabrics, so you might have to adapt certain styles to your particular shape.

If you're overweight, you could try a diet. Chances are you have tried, and you will try—but right now you're too heavy. Maybe you're permanently overweight, and maybe you're one of those people who keeps fluctuating. You don't have to buy a wardrobe of assorted sizes for pre-diet, post-diet and during diet. Instead, concentrate on the kind of loose clothing that's always attractive and always in style. I mean beautiful caftans, wonderful tunics: the long, loose flowing look that conceals without seeming to. Nobody can tell what's going on underneath—a model figure, too much sauerkraut or a five-month pregnancy.

Caftans are perfect evening wear, particularly for at-homes. They can be casual enough to wear on the beach over your bathing suit, or dressy enough for black tie occasions. You can get them in any color, and in wide range of fabrics from a simple, natural cotton to filmy chiffon to a rich silk or satin brocade. They can have some fit to them or hang loose from the shoulders, and their length can go from groin (over skirts or pants) to the floor.

If your breasts are large, you might try a caftan that fits smoothly at the sides of the breasts, or one that fits over the top of the breasts and falls in a straight line from nipples or, even better, from just above the nipples. This line is especially good for minimizing extremely large breasts.

Tunics, burnooses, djellabas and all the A-line clothes look very

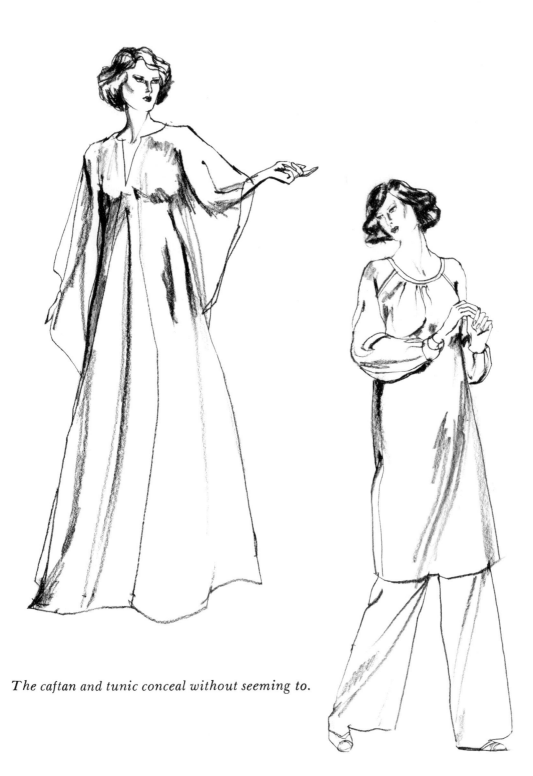

The caftan and tunic conceal without seeming to.

good on a heavy woman. Wear overblouses or loose-fitting sweaters over skirts or pants. Don't wear anything that's fussy, and run as fast as you can from a ruffle. Choose lightweight fabrics, even for winter. Thick, heavy fabrics will only emphasize your heaviness. If you wear furs, choose one with a short pile. If you're dying for that marvelous, dreamy peach-colored angora sweater, you have two choices: Either lose the excess weight, or be prepared to resemble a cute baby hippopotamus.

Your choices should be very thin wools and synthetics that hold their shape and have a light, airy feeling. Choose colors that bring out your skin tone and eyes. Avoid anything too elaborate or fussy, in the garment itself and in accessories and jewelry. If you like patterns, select one that's not too strong. You can also wear the old reliable stripes that go up and down; they'll lengthen and slim you.

If your breasts are very large, then, generally speaking, you won't look your best in suits. The jacket won't hang well on you. Suits are usually designed for the average- or small-breasted woman. If you do buy a suit, choose one with a long (even very long) jacket, preferably in a knit. The best jacket on you is quite thin and drops straight down close to the body. Any kind of box jacket is a disaster; it'll just bring out top-heaviness.

Try to emphasize your waist and balance off the weight of your breasts with fuller skirts, to establish proportion between top and bottom. Any form-fitting sheath will make you appear top-heavy; and don't wear tight sweaters or gathered tops. Extremely large breasts are not attractive, certainly not in clothes and probably not (if the truth be known) to most men either.

Before anything else, choose the right bra. It should smooth and control, bringing the breasts up high enough to look good in clothes, but not so high that they look even larger. Don't get a bra with straps that cut deeply into your flesh. Ask an experienced saleswoman for help in selecting one.

The only permanent solution for very large breasts is plastic surgery, and if your breasts are really enormous and painful, I'd suggest that you consider it. Otherwise, minimize and balance.

If you're both breasty and hippy, you have an hourglass figure, and I'm sure you don't need me to tell you to emphasize it by making your waist look as small as you can manage.

If your breasts are very small, most clothes today are designed for you, and you'll wear them much better than a large-breasted woman. All the see-throughs are for you. There's almost no style that won't work on you—even a strapless evening gown. If the dress requires more fullness, you can always supply it with a padded bra.

Audrey Hepburn, who's very small-breasted, looks perfect in almost everything. I've seen Audrey in strapless dresses and she looks divine. I don't think she does anything to add to her breast size—she just looks stunning. Whatever she wears seems made just for her. Peasant clothes, suits, gowns all look high-style on her. For Sophia Loren, on the other hand, dressing is a much tougher problem.

Women who are long-waisted and have short legs should avoid splitting up color between top and bottom. A solid look is best. If you must have a belt, wear it high, to give more length to your legs. Or go without a belt, so there's no definite waistline and the eye can't see where the legs begin. These are tricks I've used because I belong in this category.

If you're short-waisted, again the beltless look is good for you. Definitely avoid all wide belts or any cummerbund, sash or waist insert that takes you from the waist to just under your breasts. This will make you look shorter and chunkier. Empire—a wonderful style generally—is a particularly good style for you.

Petite women should wear the thinnest possible fabric and avoid layering to keep your miniature Dresden appeal. If you feel more mushroom than Dresden, stick with the most tailored clothes you can find.

Very tall women can wear almost everything, with the exception of

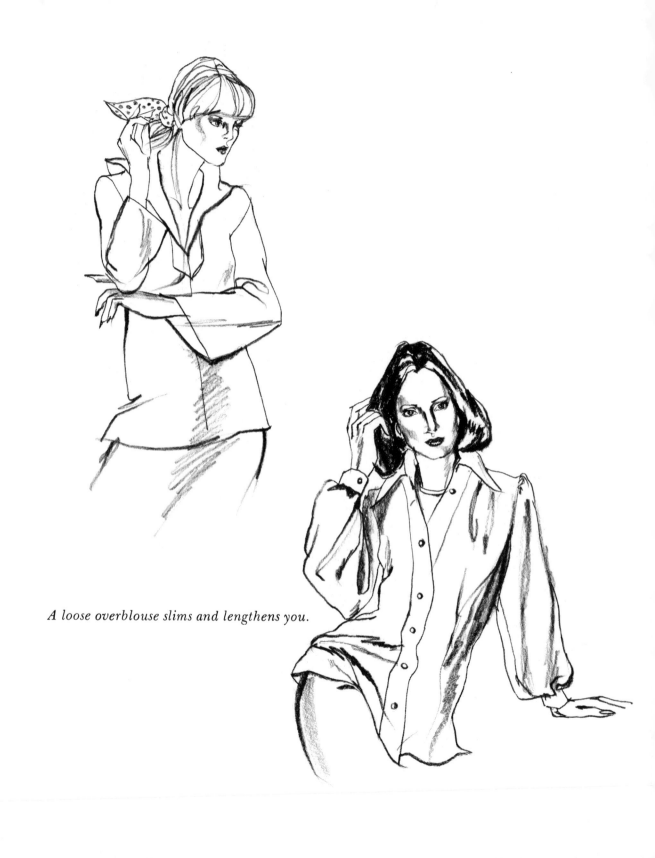

A loose overblouse slims and lengthens you.

extremely fussy or frilly clothes. The "cute" look of pinafores and other little-girl outfits is slightly ridiculous on six-footers.

If you're thin besides being tall, the fashion world is your oyster. You can wear all fabrics, all the prints, checks, stripes you want. And you, more than anyone, can go in for layering.

Most women know—or eventually learn—what flatters them and what doesn't. You may look best in very tailored clothes, in peasant dresses or perhaps in Oriental gowns. You know your best colors and styles because you've received compliments for them. Gather those compliments like suggestion slips, and pay attention to them, but most of all pay attention to how *you* feel in clothes.

I, for instance, love ascots. The double-ascot look is tremendously chic. It's a scarf double-tied, so that it goes round the neck once, comes back in front and ties in a bow or is lapped over like a man's tie. But if I wear it, I look as though my chin is resting on my shoulders. No one has to tell me—I *know* it. I also won't wear chokers. The closest I'll come is a very, very thin, almost baby-weight chain around the neck with maybe one drop pendant that falls into the hollow of the neck. Needless to say, I'm not long-necked.

If you have a short neck, always try to cheat your neckline down, just below the jewel neck. Don't wear chokers or scarves tied around the neck (no double-tied ascot, obviously), and make sure your jewelry drops. Matinée length (about thirty inches) or longer is good.

A long neck looks marvelous in a very high turtle. A normal neck can wear everything it wants around it.

These are a few known principles for minimizing defects. But the best way to distract attention from what you don't want people to notice is to play up whatever it is you do want them to see. The difference beween an optimist and a pessimist is that the pessimist believes people are noticing a large belly and chunky knees while the optimist knows people are looking at the clear eyes and smooth skin. If you plan your wardrobe like an optimist, you'll pay more attention to emphasizing

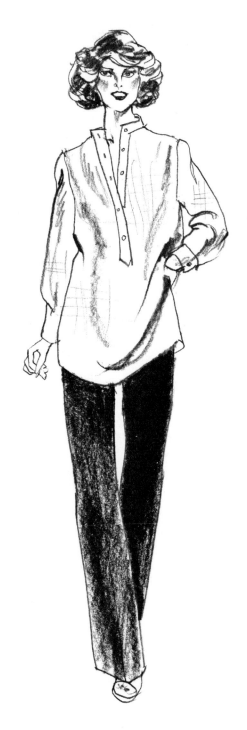

If your waist is too large or in the wrong place, go beltless.

your good qualities than to minimizing your defects. And it'll probably work. Clear eyes will be remembered much longer than chunky knees.

Dress Wise: Accessorize!

In Paradise, the fig leaf was a basic outfit; today, it would be an accessory. Accessories provide the joy, imaginativeness and creativity of dressing. They stretch out even the most meager wardrobe in all sorts of wonderful directions. They let you experiment with fashion at very low cost. They let you express your individuality. They transform a single garment or a two-piece outfit into a total look. If dressing is a statement you make about yourself, accessories are your signature.

They'll crop up throughout this book and help with every part of the body. Accessories are the secret of successful dressing for the modern woman who doesn't have time (or inclination) to go home and change her clothes for each event in her day. She starts out in the morning in a dress or suit, and she's still wearing it in the evening. By day it was businesslike, with a look of authority. In the evening, it's suddenly soft and feminine. Same dress, same woman, but she's learned to make her clothes change along with her moods. When the efficient businesswoman leaves the office, she's left one aspect of herself behind. The evening woman is different—more gentle, perhaps, more seductive or flirtatious. So are her clothes, now slightly bared or set off with jewelry, or with an emphasis created by a scarf.

Accessorizing is the most essential part of dressing, and also the most fun; it lets you be adventurous and individualistic, from head to toe.

Hats: To Wear or Not to Wear

There was a time when every woman had to own at least one hat. I had two—one for all weddings, the other for all funerals. I don't think I look good in hats, and one of the greatest things that's happened to me in fashion is that hats have gone off the list of necessities (even for weddings and funerals). A hat is not a necessity anywhere except in Vatican City or in Catholic churches—but even there, alternate headwear (kerchiefs, babushkas, mantillas) will do.

Some women were born to wear hats. There's a face for every kind of hat: flower hat and picture hat, little veiled hat; hat with a peak, wide brim, narrow brim; floppy hat, stiff hat, man's hat and even Stetson. Some women were born to wear turbans. We know who these women are, because they look terrific in them, and they carry it off with aplomb.

Others, no matter how hard they try, can't make it come off. A hat makes a very strong impression, and you need a lot of self-assurance to wear one with ease. Bella Abzug has made hats so much a projection of her very visible personality that she'd probably seem naked without one.

But as a whole, hats are being worn less and less—with the exception of beach hats, straw and raffia hats, and rain hats. They're no longer the status symbol they used to be, in the days when an executive woman might wear a hat, but her secretary wouldn't. Today, it tends to be the other way around, if anything. The executive woman, having attained a position that few women ever achieved before this time in history, feels secure enough not to have to announce her position in an obvious way. She feels free not to ever wear a hat unless it pleases her. The secretary, on the other hand, might wear one if she's trying to become an executive. The hat would give her a look of competence, style and courage.

It wouldn't do that for me. Some women will always look silly in a hat, turban or even a babushka. I come very close to being one of them. I have nothing against hats, and I sometimes have an urge to try again, especially when I see a girl in a fashion magazine wearing a bathing suit or caftan, with a wonderfully wrapped turban on her head. Or she's wearing a dressier, just-as-wonderful turban in a fancy restaurant. Or she's out dancing, with a crazy little veil on her head that she needs courage to wear. But I can't even wrap a turban properly, though I've been taught by experts. I guess my will just isn't in it. Somehow or other I realize this isn't for me.

If you want to wear a hat, and you're looking for that one classic that goes with everything, your best bet is a fedora. Get it in the right kind of fabric—a light, thin felt or velvet—and you can change it from a day hat to an evening hat by taking off the grosgrain band and replacing it with a dressier band of satin or brocade. One fedora with a number of hat bands can be the hat for all occasions. Instead of a band, you might even try the look that's always new one year, old the next, then new again; I mean Indian beading.

If you love hats, and want to wear them at every possible opportunity, do. There are many occasions when hats are suitable, though by no means required, and these are indicated throughout the book.

How to Make Scarves Work for You

There are other things you can put on your head besides hats. In winter you'll want woolly caps to keep you warm—bright knitted cloches or colorful crochets. In a church, you can wear a lace mantilla, laid gently on the top of your head and flowing down. You can wear flowers in your hair, and ribbons, and tiaras and other jewelry for the head. But, no matter what else you do or don't wear, you'll be certain to need scarves.

Today scarves come in all sizes, colors and practically every material. They are worn on different parts of the body as accessories or as garments in themselves. But let's start at the top, with a cotton or silk (or synthetic) square that you wear over your head. You wear it for fashion, fun or protection—sometimes for all three. It protects your hair from wind and rain. It conceals hair that's in need of shampoo or,

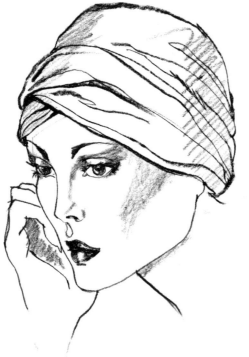

Some women were born to wear turbans, others fedoras.

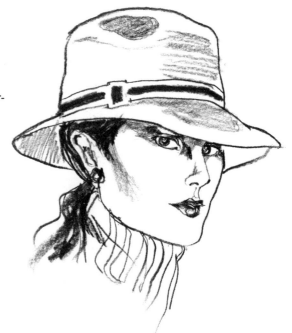

when the roots are showing, a color touch-up. You wear it to keep hair out of your face when you're sailing or engaging in other outdoor sports. You wear it to keep the sun off (particularly for artificially colored hair) in summer.

As a fashion item, it can be tied or bound in a number of ways to suit your face. It sets off your outfit with color, or is of the same material as something else you're wearing. Many cotton sundresses are now being sold with a matching square just large enough to cover your shoulders, or ample for your head, to achieve an ensemble look.

Fashion dictates new ways to tie a scarf every season but I suggest that you choose the way that looks best on you and suits what you're wearing. With very informal clothes, shorts and jeans, and with peasant-type clothes, a babushka tied under the chin looks just right. At the same time, this look will slim down a large or round face.

If you have a thin or long face, you might look better with the scarf tied at the back of your head. Or wear it Aunt Jemima style. You can twist the ends in back and curl it into a chignon for a very sleek look. Caribbeans have wonderful, complicated ways of tying and pinning scarves so they look like elaborate headdresses. It won't hurt to experiment. Try moving the scarf down on your forehead, with no hair showing. Keep moving it back and bring out your hair, until you have it positioned at the best place for you.

When you're wearing a scarf around the neck, you again have a variety of choices. For the head, use large or small squares (oblongs for turbans), but for the neck, small squares or oblongs. Tie the scarf loosely or lightly around the neck for a choker, or knot it a few inches lower for a cowl effect. Let it be an ascot, once- or twice-tied around the neck; or wear it like a man's tie or bow tie.

You'll need a large shawl or stole for your shoulders. Large triangles are good, and so are long scarves. The old fur stole is out, so if you buy a fur for your shoulders, make sure it's really a long scarf. Cashmere and thin wool shawls are excellent. If you crochet, spend some winter

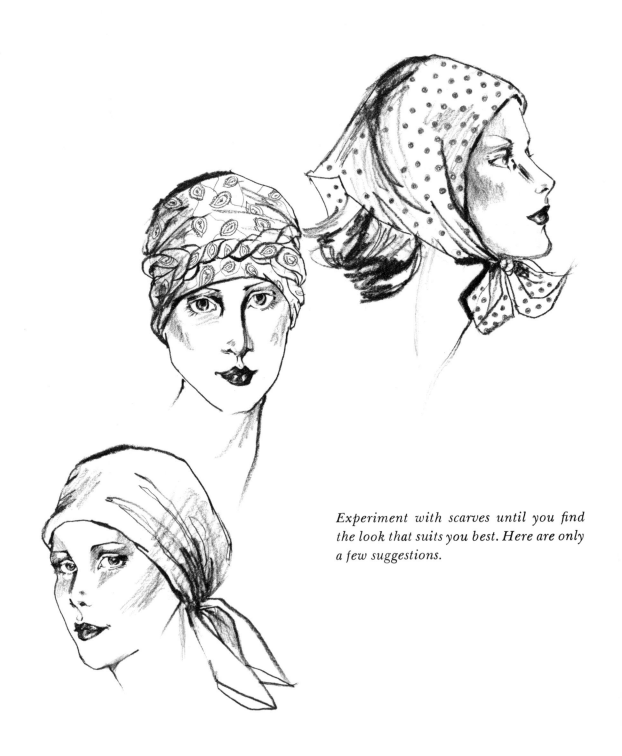

Experiment with scarves until you find the look that suits you best. Here are only a few suggestions.

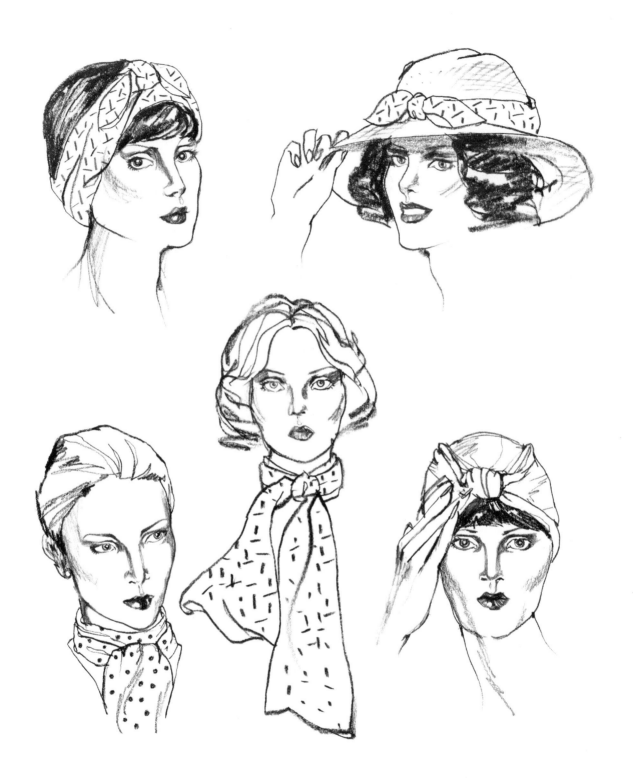

hours whipping up a frothy, lacy summer stole. Satin and silk stoles are perfect for dressing up an outfit. A very, very long thin silk stole can be draped over any simple dress and turn it into something spectacular.

Under the breasts (the Empire style), at the waist or on the hips, scarves become belts, sashes, cummerbunds, even skirts or blouses. They can be as wide or as narrow as you like, with a single tie, a bow, a knot or pinned on. Take a long scarf with a fringe, tie it around your waist, let the fringe hang down—and you have a very dressy look.

A scarf can move throughout the day, from the neck, where it may be concealing a low-cut blouse, to become a sash around the waist in the evening. Tied low on the chest, it gives a sexy look to the most tailored suit in the world worn without a blouse.

If it's large enough, a scarf can be a skirt, a fanny-hugger, a long skirt, even a long sundress (wrapped around the breasts at the top). It can go over skirts, dresses or pants for the layered look. A smaller scarf can be a summer top—anything from a strapless bra to a halter to a covered front with bare back.

Even if you're not wearing it, a scarf can add to the total look of your outfit when you tie it around the strap of your handbag. It's there to give an element of color, and if there's a sudden rain, you can put it over your head. Skiers can add to their look by tying a scarf around the top of their ski pole, or on the strap.

Just as you can never be too thin or too rich, you also can't have too many scarves. More than any other accessory, they can update and extend any wardrobe. They're the ideal way to experiment with a color you've never worn before. Whatever size or shape they are, you'll definitely be able to use them—*some* place.

Jewelry: Restraint Is a Girl's Best Friend

Jewelry is the oldest accessory known to man or woman and is worn in all cultures, even those that have no use for clothes. Wear jewelry

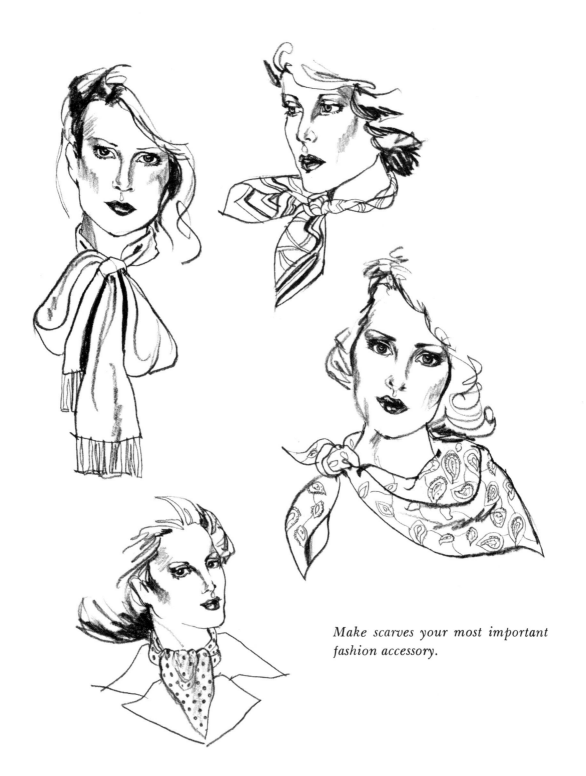

Make scarves your most important fashion accessory.

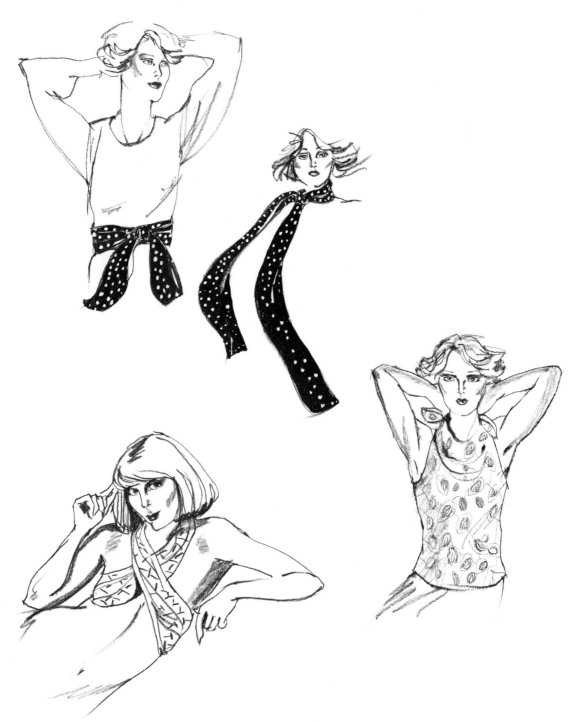

Let your imagination run wild—be dramatic, sexy, colorful.

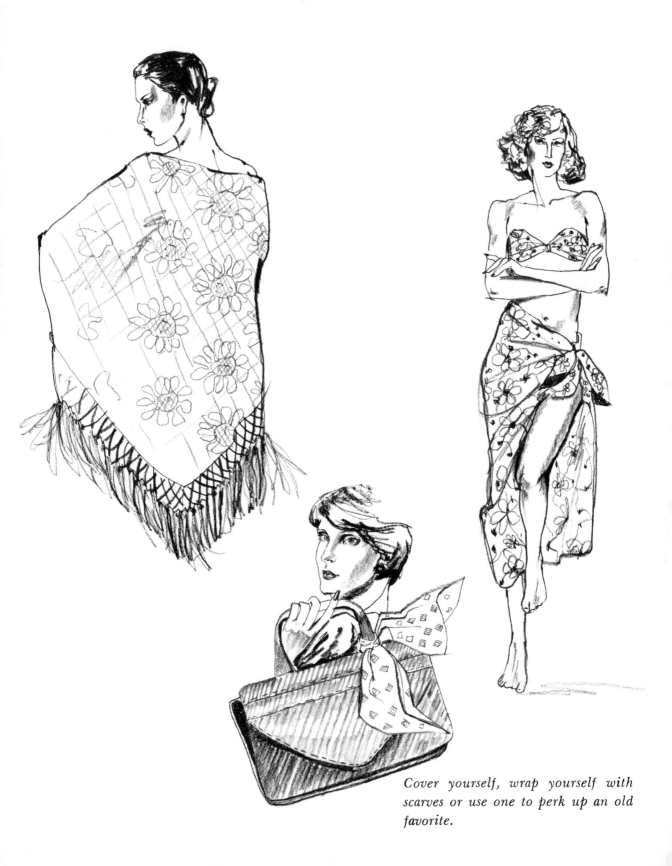

Cover yourself, wrap yourself with scarves or use one to perk up an old favorite.

of whatever design you like, and let it be real or costume, but never wear too much. Any very large piece of jewelry should probably be the only piece you wear. Let it then be the focus of your outfit: a wonderful brooch on your shoulder or hip; a broad gleaming necklace; exquisite long drop earrings. Never wear a large necklace with large or long earrings. Each distracts from the other and gives you a cluttered look.

Keep simplicity as your motto. The wonderful piece you inherited from your grandmother shouldn't have to compete with anything else. On the other hand, if you're wearing thin chains, you can wear a number of them without looking fussy. The same is true of bracelets and, sometimes, rings.

Jewelry is not strictly part of clothing. You're on your own with it. Just remember it should add to whatever else you're wearing, not be distracting. Excessive jewelry always means overdressing. If that's your weakness, follow the rule to always remove one piece of jewelry before you go out.

Other Accessories

Handbags are covered in Chapter 3 along with briefcases. (See "In the Business Bag.")

What belts can do for you

Belts can add variety to an outfit, and update it. If you have clothes you've owned for years, a new belt will change the effect. Go from a narrow belt to a wide one, or vice versa; from a matching- to contrasting-color belt; from a waist to hip belt.

Shoes: Comfort comes first

When you're buying shoes, try to find an acceptable ground between fashion and comfort. Don't buy plastic shoes studded with rhinestones unless you're going to appear in the revival of an old musical. Shoes

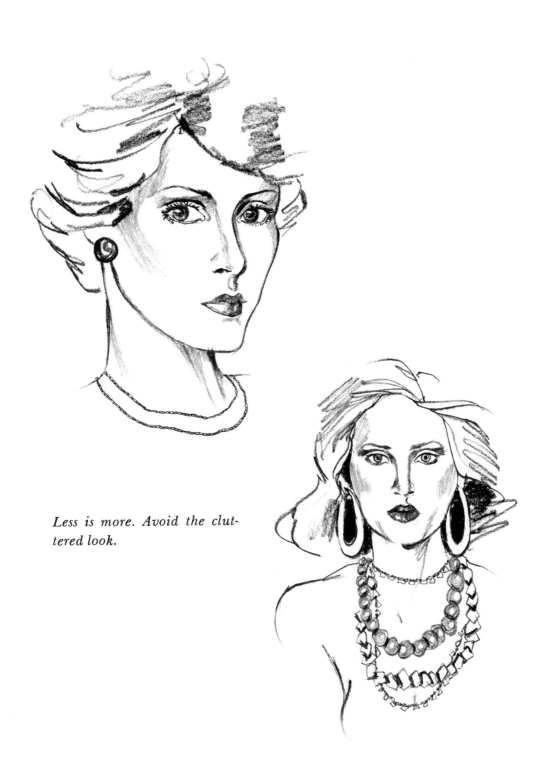

Less is more. Avoid the clut-tered look.

dyed to match a dress or bag are out. If a shoe store is offering fantastic discounts on five-inch stilettoes left over from the fifties, ignore them.

Shoes used to provide instant torture for millions of women. They were too tight at some part of the foot, you never felt safe wearing them, they threw the body out of line and caused waves of backaches, not to mention aching feet. Also, women were indoctrinated in a kind of suicidal vanity that said small feet were better than big feet. So you tried to squeeze your size seven into a six, and the shoe salesman helped your effort by bringing out sizes smaller than the one your foot measured.

I don't think many women do that anymore. It's absolutely crazy, besides being uncomfortable and unhealthy. Don't stick to the size you've always worn, either. Feet can grow or swell, particularly in summer. My feet have increased in size over the years. It's best always to have your feet measured when you're buying shoes, and then to get the proper size.

A heel of some kind looks best on most women. It lengthens and slims your legs and improves your posture. A flat heel tends to make you slouch. However, if you're six feet tall and don't want to add to your height through heels, get flat shoes and tell yourself to stand up straight. But I've noticed that many women who are six feet or over still choose small heels. The added inch or two is less important to them than looking chic.

Don't go in the other direction, either—to five- or six-inch heels. They'll make you walk in a strange way, and when people offer you their arm, it's more likely to be due to the impulse of a good Samaritan than romance or passion.

Your basic shoe wardrobe should consist of two pairs for daytime wear, evening slippers, a pair of sandals, bedroom slippers, and a pair of boots or good, solid walking shoes that won't melt in the rain. If you invest in a pair of good black leather shoes for daytime wear, they'll take you into most evenings.

Go easy on gloves

Like hats, gloves used to be on the necessities list, and are now off it. Formerly a woman without gloves was simply not well-dressed. Today, a woman with gloves is almost an oddity—unless she's meeting royalty.

Gloves should be worn for warmth in winter, and for any sport that requires them. I wear gloves for bike riding, and some people find them comfortable for driving. Otherwise, I wear gloves only for really formal events, and then they're the long three- or six-button kind. They are imperative only for a white-tie-and-tails affair.

For most women, a pair of fur- or cashmere-lined leather gloves and a pair of wool gloves are enough, with perhaps an additional pair of black or white leather gloves for formal winter evenings.

Europeans wear gloves more than we do, so you might take along a pair of white glacé ones for the opera when you travel. But generally, gloves have gone from being essential to optional. And in casual situations, they're definitely *de trop*.

Accessorizing is an art in itself, an elaboration on the art of dressing, with fewer risks. There's no way you can make really big mistakes with accessories, unless you put on too many at the same time. To the meat of dressing, they are the sauce; to the cake, the icing.

When It's Raining . . .

have no regrets. Rainwear can be a stunning part of your wardrobe. You can go in almost any direction with it now; it's exciting and fun. Rain suits, for example, are chic and practical. I have two, each a three-piece outfit with skirt, jacket and pants. One is in khaki with a wraparound skirt. It looks like a regular suit or pantsuit, but is of rainproof material. The other is of a very, very thin rain fabric, almost like a windbreaker. It's definitely intended for rain, but it looks smashing.

On days when rain has been predicted, or when it's actually pouring outside, it's great to own a suit like one of these because you can go anywhere without looking like a drowned rat who's thrown a raincoat over everything. It's chic, fun, interesting to have, and serves well for many occasions.

Raincoats now come in all styles, in a variety of fabrics and colors. You can get a cape, a loose belted coat, a poncho or any other style you wish in lengths going from short jacket to long coat. If you're investing in a large rain wardrobe, get anything that pleases you, but if you have only one raincoat—and you *must* own one—make it traditional. The trench coat is very attractive and looks good on just about everyone, but it can get too warm in the summer. I love the loose type of raincoat that's almost a duster and will double as a summer coat.

It's a wonderful item to own: a very lightweight coat in a light silky material with a loose body that goes over everything. It can be very dressy but doesn't look out of place over pants, is great for evening wear, over lounging pajamas, a long dinner dress or over a dressy long skirt and blouse. It gives you an additional thin, dressy coat.

It's also perfect over suits or a day dress. I'd like every woman to own one. It'll take her through spring, summer and fall as a coat and as a raincoat.

In winter, I rarely wear a raincoat. I wear winter coats with a large umbrella and rain boots. I'll wear furs in the rain and I don't worry. After all, these furs ran around in rain and snow when they were alive, and it didn't hurt them—so it seems only fair that rain and snow shouldn't hurt them when they're coats.

If, however, you have a really wonderful fur, like a chinchilla or broadtail or sable, and you don't want to take chances, you can get one of the new extra-large-size rain covers or capes to put over the fur.

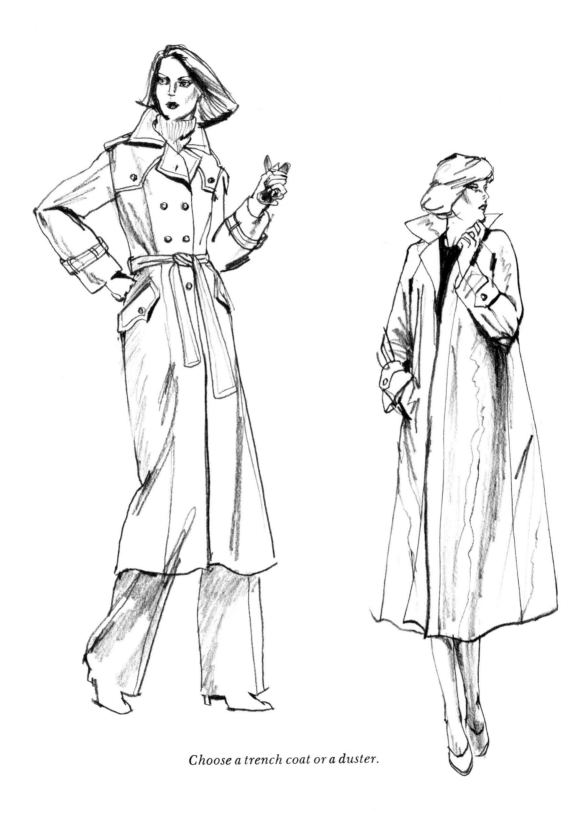

Choose a trench coat or a duster.

It will protect the coat completely, and looks as though you're wearing a trench coat lined with fur.

If you're buying a lined raincoat, get one with removable lining so you'll be able to wear it in warmer weather. If the lining is fur, you'll want to remove it for summer storage.

Rain hats, like coats, come in a great variety of styles. If you look good in hats and enjoy wearing them, get a rain hat in the style that's most becoming to you. If you don't usually wear hats, you can get sporty caps to protect your hair and keep the rain off your face, and they'll look terrific.

Get the kind of windjammer boating cap that goes with a slicker. It's what the captain of an old fishing trawler would wear, and is a wonderfully attractive, slouchy kind of hat that really, honestly keeps the rain off.

Or buy yourself a newsboy's oversized cap with a visor or bill that deflects the rain from your face. It's large enough for you to push all your hair into it, and you can be sure your hair will stay totally dry. When you take off the cap, you shake your hair into shape. The cap is roomy enough not to crush it.

If you hate hats on all occasions, get a rain babushka. It can be a treated material in bright colors, or even a plastic bonnet, almost a hairnet of transparent plastic. It costs practically nothing and is perfect for carrying along in case of rain or drizzle. If you always have it with you, you never have to wear a special hat for rain. It'll go directly over your hair, or over the scarf or turban you're wearing.

Boots are wonderful in the rain—any kind of boots, from treated leather to rubber. Treated leather, however, is usually only rain-resistant, not waterproof. It's fine for drizzle or light rain, but won't hold up in puddles. If you're wearing good shoes or evening slippers, you'll have to get overshoes in plastic or rubber.

Rain no longer means that you have to look dowdy. You don't have to put on old clothes or cancel an appointment because you have

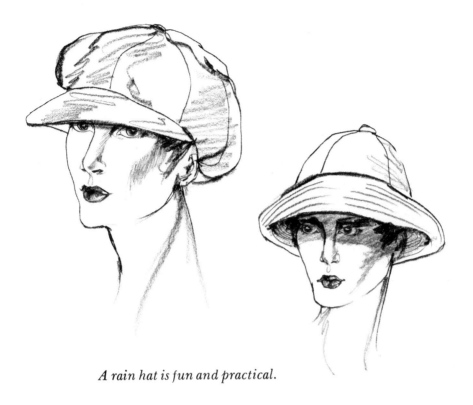

A rain hat is fun and practical.

nothing to wear. Put on your rain suit, or your favorite dress with the duster over it, wear a smile on your face, pin a bunch of violets on your coat and laugh at the clouds.

Underneath It All

One function of clothing is to conceal defects of the body. It conceals, but doesn't correct. No clothing in the world will give you a sensational figure if you don't have one to begin with—and the better your figure, the more choice you'll have in what to wear, and the better your clothes will look on you.

I'd Love To, But What'll I Wear?

Women with the tall, lean body of a model, with long legs and average-to-small breasts, will look good in almost everything, including potato sacks. They're the lucky ones, who can buy the least expensive clothing and still look like a million.

Women who are overweight, or have any particular figure problem, will have to invest more time and money in their clothes if they want to look chic. They have to hunt for that skirt with a little more give to it, for the very long jacket, for the long dress in a material that holds its own and drops gracefully to the floor.

Twenty years ago women bought heavily constructed undergarments to hold them in, flatten them out, push them up or smooth them down. Girdles were very tight and strong, corsets were boned, and if you didn't like the way you looked from neck to thigh, you could always choose a total foundation.

I think the constructed look has gone for good, along with the very heavy makeup, the thick pancake foundation. The severely controlled body was never sexy, and now it's not elegant either. Clothes are much softer than they were, fabrics more supple and clinging. To see the outline of whalebones or the seam of brassiere through a soft knit is far more off-putting than seeing the outline of a breast.

Ideally, I feel that a woman should actively do something to improve the shape she's in. I suggest diets and exercise instead of girdles and corsets. As our life-style has changed in the past twenty years, so has our way of dressing. In 1957 girls wore Merry Widow bras under their tulle prom dresses; in 1977, they're more likely to be braless under a thin knit or even gauze.

Our life-style is easier, and women particularly are much freer than they used to be. Sex, in and out of marriage, is much more open. And women, out of their houses much more than they used to be, are busy at all kinds of activities and jobs.

The woman of the seventies is a feminine *person*. Her appearance shows who she is and what she does while never losing sight of the

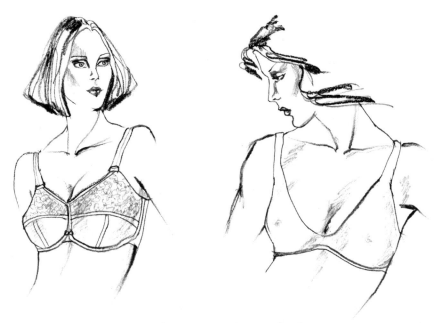

Choose the bra your figure requires.

fact that she's a woman. (Men are making the same kind of statement, with their unconstructed jackets and body shirts.)

Try to do without controlling garments as much as possible. If you need to conceal, wear loose clothes over underwear that's lightly constructed. Support hose will lightly hold in fanny, thighs and hips without an iron maiden look. Body stockings are excellent, particularly if flesh colored under sheer clothes, to give the impression of a chaste nudity. You won't look naked, but you'll appear much freer than if you wear a slip. Try to get body stockings with garters attached, so they won't creep up behind.

Bras are highly personal, the most personal of all garments. Choose the style that gives you the best line and is most comfortable. That means selecting the bra with the least construction you can get away with. However, if you need underwiring, padding or side control, get it.

In a strapless bra, go by your own preference. Some women are comfortable in short ones—others feel constricted and prefer a longer line.

As a general rule, just keep away from highly constructed undergarments as much as you can. You have a chance now to be a freer, more comfortable woman than you ever were—so take it.

Tots to Teens

As every mother knows, the little darlings can be impossible when it comes to dress. Particularly if they're boys. You ask them to put on a clean pair of pants or a suit, and the siege begins. Hours later you may have won, but the victory doesn't seem worth it. The child is properly dressed, but the expression on his face is sour as a trumpet player sucking lemons.

My two girls have a very good style of dressing, I feel, but my teen-age son is not interested. Clothes don't matter to him—yet. In another year or so we may all be fighting for the mirror, but now the last thing in the world that interests him is clothes.

I pretty well know my son's attitude to dressing, and I try to adapt to it. I know that if I make a lunch or dinner reservation for the two of us someplace where he has to wear a suit and tie, the hassle I'll have to go through for hours is not worth it to me. I don't want to lose those hours of my life in aggravation. Instead, I'll deliberately seek out a restaurant where he can dress in a way that makes him comfortable.

Of course there are times when you have to tell a child what to wear, and force him to comply or leave him home. You don't want to (and there's no reason why you should have to) show up at a wedding followed by scruffy children. Parents must guide children in dressing, and at the same time help them to develop their style. I find the best method is to give your children an enormous amount of freedom to make their own statement and then, in a noncritical way, let them know whether their statement works or not.

You start training your children from birth, whether you're aware of it or not. Your own attitudes will carry through to them, and it's important to know what they are.

The baby is born. You carry your pride home from the hospital and shortly afterward you prepare for his or her viewing by friends and relations. It's fine for you to get that one gorgeous, extravagant "the-baby's-on-display" outfit, but only one. Anything more is silly—those beautiful items won't be worn. The baby isn't a doll, but a living creature who will soil the frills and laces and not look as cute as you'd like when his small face is bright red with indignation. Little jumpers, the terry one-pieces, diaper covers and short shirts are all an infant needs, and all that a mother should have to care for.

Now the baby is crawling, walking, gurgling or talking. Cute as a button, the cleverest baby in the world, and it's almost impossible to resist showing him off. You want all the adorable little things to put on him or her. But remember that children grow extremely quickly. An outfit will go from much too large to small or to unwearable in months, and it probably won't even be worn during the snippet of time when it fits perfectly. A child will wear it once or twice, so unless you're planning a large family and count on handing down the little velvet suits and frilly dresses, don't buy them.

A large investment in children's clothing is outrageous. You'll probably be given beautiful little things by godparents, grandparents, friends and others who can't resist. Beautiful little baby things are marvelous to look at, the greatest fun in the world to shop for, a joy to buy, but very expensive and impractical.

When the child reaches school age—anywhere from nursery school through grade school—the gorgeous, extravagant items should be limited to one at a time. (Even so, you can end up buying a dozen or more such items as the child outgrows one after another.) And that one, however divine, fluffy and fabulous it is, should still be machine washable. Most American baby and children's clothes are, but read the label in any case, and beware of imports.

Let your children wear clothes they can live in comfortably. You set up a psychological problem for your children when you dress them for yourself, to show off. The outfit becomes too important. At times it seems the outfit is more important than the child, so you shout, "Don't get that dress dusty!" or you yell, "Watch out! You're getting mud on your pants leg."

This is an almost guaranteed way to turn the child off clothes, off dressing. You're really saying to the child: "When you're dressed, don't be comfortable." That's the effect of the training you're giving, and you'll learn to regret it.

If you want your child to have a special outfit for visitors, let him know exactly what its purpose is. Even if the child will later say, "This is my show-me-off-to-Grandma outfit," that's O.K. Grandma will probably laugh, and the child is getting an honest sense of what clothes are all about.

It's best for you and your children if you train them from the very beginning to enjoy what they wear, to know they can have fun in clothes—and at the same time to give them a sense of taking care of their clothes, though not to the point of yelling at them whenever you see a particle of dust.

When I was a little girl, I adored clothes. Though my parents didn't have much money, this was the one area in which they really indulged me. I owned every Shirley Temple dress that was ever made. Sometimes I'd give away my dresses, if other little girls admired them. I was permitted to wear my dresses to school, and that made sense. If a child doesn't wear the clothes everywhere, they'll be outgrown before they're worn.

If I had a little girl today who wanted to dress the way I did as a child, I'd take her choice seriously and talk to her honestly about it:

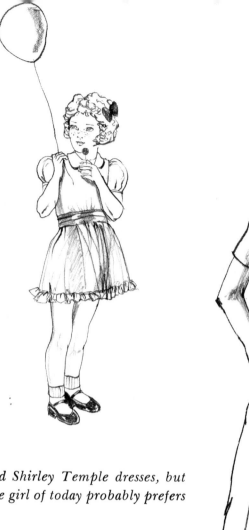

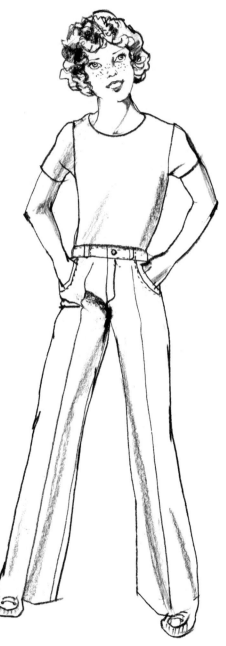

I adored Shirley Temple dresses, but the little girl of today probably prefers jeans.

"It's lovely that you want to wear frilly little dresses, and I'll get one for you if it's really what you'd prefer. But you'll have to be responsible for the dress. I'll get you one of those, and I'll also get you pants and tops and crazy colored socks. On the days when you want to be a perfect little lady, you'll wear your frilly dress. You won't be able to play too much in the playground or do any roughhousing because you might tear or soil the dress. On the days when you want to cut up, climb the jungle gym and ride down the slides, you'll wear the pants."

This way, you're giving the child the possibility of choice, and at the same time you're teaching her to be responsible. You may be surprised by how seriously the child will then take her responsibility. You're proposing an exchange, and she realizes you're being fair.

I pick out clothes for my children and shop for them. But when they reach a certain age, you have to realize you can't force your taste on them—not in today's society. At one time you not only could, you did. When I was little, my mother would say, "You wear that," and I'd answer, "Yes, ma'am." That's what I wore and there simply wasn't any discussion about it.

Today, if you try that line on a child past the third grade, there is probably going to be trouble. The child will rebel, and you'll have hours of haranguing and aggravation on your hands. If you shop for children and go only by what you like, you simply might be throwing your money away. The child will ignore the half a dozen new pants you bought in a style that none of his playmates wear and instead will every day get into the old torn ones you hoped to replace.

Realize you'll have to end up buying what *they* want, though of course there are limits. You'll also have to ensure they have a basic wardrobe. Each year I buy my son a suit, which, if I'm lucky, he'll wear once before he outgrows it, and that one wearing will probably be at all but the threat of death. I'll have to cajole, vow to lock him in his room for a week, or whatever, to get him to put it on. Yet it's necessary for that particular occasion.

The Joy of Clothing

If you plan on giving your child a clothes allowance—and it's a marvelous idea—wait until he or she is fifteen. Unless your child has a precocious sense of clothes, he won't be competent to handle a clothes allowance earlier. And start by giving an allowance for little things only: underwear, stockings, combs, brushes—essential items.

Don't be too critical of what the child selects, either when he's with you or on his own. He knows what the other children are wearing and will probably want to conform. That sense of safety is necessary for his growing up. I think every parent should visit his child's school at least once to see what other children are wearing. Your child is being exposed to peer pressure every day. Children can be very cruel, and if you force your child to dress differently from the others, he may be teased for it and suffer needlessly.

When children grow older and start to move away from conformity, encourage them. Expose them to magazines and give them leeway to develop individuality in dressing. This is particularly essential for the private school or parochial school child who has to wear a uniform every day. That uniform can stifle individuality, so it's very important that your child be able to dress as he likes when he comes home.

Don't make fun of your children's clothing choices or put them down. Don't go by the rules we had to follow when we were kids—they don't exist anymore. We were warned *never* to wear red and purple together; today, it's one of the most popular color combinations. The clothes I wore when I was a kid would seem ridiculous now: the fluffy, organdy dress with a big sash to tie in the back, ribbons in the hair, white bobby socks and Mary Jane patent leather shoes. I adored all of it, but most little girls today wouldn't be caught dead in such an outfit. We led different lives then; today's little girl may be an out-fielder in the Little League. She might long for a catcher's mitt, a doctor's uniform or an astronaut's outfit.

I remember wanting a nurse's uniform more than anything else. When I was eight or nine you could send away for one as a bonus after you'd sold so many jars of Clovereen salve. The uniform consisted of a white apron and a white nurse's cap. That was it, but to me it was the most exciting, necessary thing I'd ever dreamed of in my life. I ordered tons of the salve, but had a very hard time selling it. So I went into a bar with my wares, and the customers bought everything I had with me. It was wonderful—they were all so happy in there, and glowing, and laughing. But my mother found out and got really angry. She made me stop going to bars, and I couldn't sell all my Clovereen salve. I never got the nurse's uniform.

Most people can remember some article of clothing that they wanted when they were children, or that they had and treasured. Even a young child can fall in love with clothes. For that reason, it's a bad idea to give children hand-me-downs. If you can possibly afford not to, don't. Parents who don't care how their children feel about a garment and are dictatorial about clothing can stifle the child's individuality.

Young children must be guided, and all children must be helped with their clothes. You'll both be happiest if you, the parent, can find a happy medium between your child's choice and what you think is appropriate. Let the child feel comfortable and not out of place among peers. Give your child leeway to make his own statement. You may be pleasantly surprised to find him saying what you hoped he'd say, and that his appearance is a source of pride to you.

A sense of clothing develops as early as a sense of self. From the moment you wrap your baby in a blanket to take him home, you're transmitting to your child your own sense of values and your attitudes. As he gets older, he'll learn from his peers also. As he changes his views, his style of dressing will change, and by the time your child is a parent he will be making a strong statement about who he is.

You start learning at birth how to compromise between your individuality and what your society expects. You learn to make a statement about who you are while at the same time being suitably dressed for the occasion.

2

Dressing for the Occasion

---

*Mr. and Mrs. Franklin Clark
request the pleasure of your company
at the wedding of their daughter
Jean
to Robert C. Guerevitch
on Saturday, June 15, 11:00 A.M.*

Weddings

After you decide on the groom, the second hardest decision is the dress. Though you may never wear it again, you'll be in it forever, young and glowing, in wedding pictures on your parents' piano and imprinted on the memories of all who were there. After your lips have tenderly told him, "Yes," your mind starts screaming: "What'll I wear?" This is one day you definitely don't want to turn up in the wrong outfit. It's unlikely that you'll have very many chances to correct your mistake.

When I was first married, at the age of eighteen and a half, would you believe that I wore a strapless white cocktail dress? I'd never been to a wedding and didn't know that brides didn't wear strapless dresses.

59

Of course it was white, but that's about as far as it went in appropriateness.

Now let me say, I do not recommend a white strapless dress for a wedding, particularly if you're the bride. But what to wear? If you're the bride, there are a variety of ways to go. And your first steps should be in the direction of the bridal shop in any major department store. Or, if you can afford it, go to the one dressmaker in town who makes the wedding dresses for "everyone." Thumb through magazines to get a sense of the type dress you'd like, and the kind of feeling you want to have at your wedding. What kind of a wedding will it be? Do you want a wonderful country-style wedding? This, I confess, is my favorite —the old-fashioned romantic wedding, with light billowing skirts and the freshness of a forest after rain, with country flowers on a mossy lawn and girls in long peasant dresses as in a country garden party of long ago.

If you choose this type of wedding, try for the tiny-church-in-the-north-of-England look, keeping everything pale and fresh. You will wear a beautiful long wedding dress in a peasant style, made of the thinnest, most delicate fabric with eyelet perhaps, or appliquéd flowers. You might add a sheer apron to it, or just the ruffles, to give it an aprony look. On your feet, wear light linen or peau de soie ballet slippers in white, or dyed to match the color of your stockinged foot.

If you decide on a veil, it should be a peasant type, though no veil is actually needed. Instead, you can entwine wonderful white flowers in your hair—lilies of the valley and baby's breath, the little buds and blossoms peeking through the strands. You'll carry a bouquet of the same flowers trailing down the front of your dress with ribbons, your diaphanous skirt touched with the green leaves of the flowers.

Your bridesmaids will be in long peasant dresses too, in a light, gauzy fabric like voile or organza. You can choose the dresses in a single color or in sheer floral print. If you can get the print in different color combinations that blend with each other, they can look like a

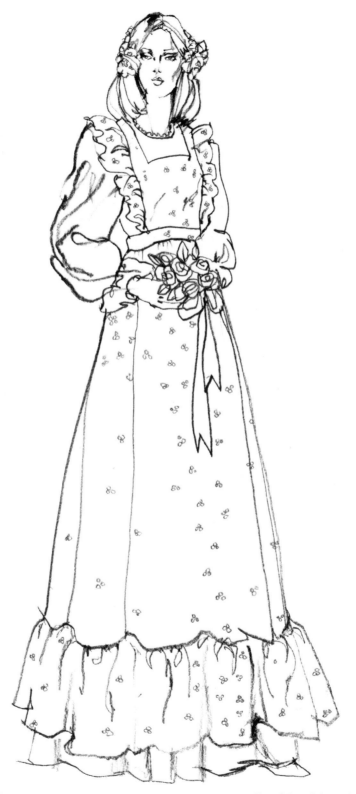

The country-style wedding dress is wonderfully old-fashioned.

bed of spring flowers. A word of warning: If there is too much contrast, if each bridesmaid is in a different dress, you'll get a cluttered look that detracts from the bride. But if you choose two or three color combinations of the exact same dress in the same print, you can achieve a beautiful orchestration with subtle variations on a theme.

The bridesmaids, too, will wear sprigs of flowers in their hair or little babushkas tied under the chin. In the latter case, you would wear a more elaborate babushka, a dreamy kerchief in lacy eyelet.

The mother of the bride, in this garden of country flowers, should wear a dress that is understated and beautfully cut. No heavy fabrics for her either, no taffetas or brocades, but she doesn't have to stick with the cottons. She can wear a dull satin, a light wool or a simple lace, in the palest green of hothouse orchids or the subtle pink of an ocean at sunset; in a faint mauve or mother-of-pearl color. Her dress should be very covered, preferably high-necked and long-sleeved, though the arms can be gauzy or translucent. And no matter what present fashion says, the dress must come to at least below her knees. Anything from there down to the floor is her decision—whatever she feels best in.

If you're invited to such a wedding, whether it's held in a church or on a rolling lawn, here is your one perfect chance to wear what used to be called "the garden tea dress." You remember that dress, don't you? It's outrageously romantic and wonderfully flattering to almost every woman. It's light and pastel, or a pale washed floral, with a wide band at the waist. It's often worn with a big picture hat, and if it suits you, by all means wear one.

For this kind of wedding, a dirndl-type or Mexican wedding dress is also perfect. Or a long, full skirt, gathered or puckered, and an embroidered vest. For the country-style wedding, let your appearance be romantic, dreamy, with a long-ago-and-far-away feeling. Maybe one of the ushers will turn out to be charming, even if he isn't a prince.

If the invitation says "black tie," chances are it's a traditional formal wedding, with Alençon lace, tiny pearls and wedding presents in crystal

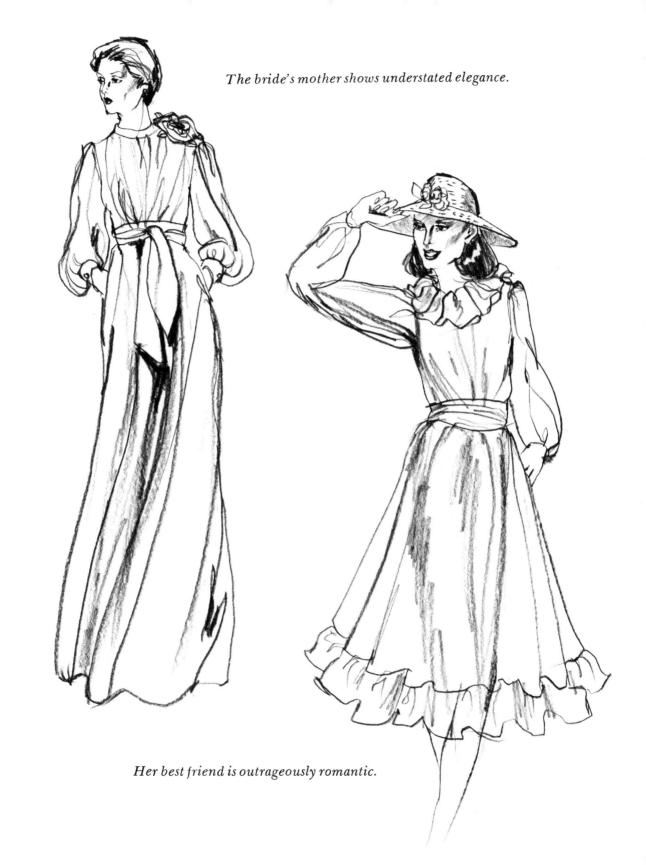

The bride's mother shows understated elegance.

Her best friend is outrageously romantic.

and silver. It will probably take place in a church or synagogue, though it could take place at home (particularly if her home is a castle).

Though the country wedding, with the bride in a long dress, is formal, this—what I call the church-church wedding—is most formal of all. Guests should wear dinner dresses or dinner suits. Even if the wedding is at eleven in the morning, do turn day to night and wear what you'd put on for a dinner party. No matter what time of day this wedding is held, it's going to be dressy. It's going to be done to the teeth.

This is your chance to shine in the daytime. You can wear any color at all, with the possible exception of white. The bride should be the only person who wears white to the wedding. If you want to express your sentiments by wearing black—go ahead. You may not be pleased by certain looks the bride and her mother send your way, but if black suits you, wear it.

If you're going to the reception only, and not to the ceremony, then black is definitely acceptable. For an evening reception where men's dress is designated as black tie (or dark suit), you have leeway between a cocktail dress and a long dinner gown or long formal gown. Avoid pants. They're inappropriate unless the bride is not wearing a long gown. And even then, only a dressy pants outfit will do.

If you want to wear a sensational, knockout cut-out dress to a wedding reception, fine. In fact, it's a terrific idea if the bridegroom has a lot of usher friends who are single. But if you're showing a lot of bare skin anywhere except in the décolleté, you're taking a chance that you'll be spotted for what you probably are, which is a lady on the prowl for an available guy. It depends on how obvious you want to be. If you don't care, or if the situation is desperate (if it's the only chance to meet all these single guys, for instance), then dare it and bare it. But stop short of the navel: A bare midriff is OK, a navel has no business being out at a wedding reception.

The bride who decides on a church-church wedding (even if it's not in a church) will wear a long white or ivory gown in satin, with tiny seed pearls or a touch of crystal decoration. The gown may have a very heavy lace trimming, and can be in any traditional cut. Brides who plan to lose thirty pounds before the Big Day would be well-advised to chose an Empire style, just in case they don't. With such a gown, the bride wears a beautiful, elaborate veil or white lace mantilla.

Her bridesmaids should be in gowns of solid colors, in taffeta or any of the dressier fabrics one step down from satin. Lace might work, though a different fabric with a tiny trim of lace would be better. The color—same for all bridesmaids—should be pastel. Prints are out.

Bride and bridesmaids will all carry flowers that have never seen a meadow or forest. The wildflower feeling of a country wedding is replaced by the elegance of lilies or white roses.

The mother of the bride in this wedding basically dresses as she would for the country wedding, though the fabric may be richer. She stays with the pale colors—beige, gray, café au lait, gray-blue, peach— but the dress is more apt to be long, and in satin or brocade. She can wear a slightly lower neckline, though a moderate scooped neck is as far as even the most glamorous mother should go, and the long sleeves remain.

Her shoes, like the bride's, should be dyed to match the gown. This is the *only* time I recommend dyeing to match, and even for this occasion a satin slipper in flesh color (the actual color of your flesh) can be worn. Since most items that are called "flesh-colored" are really the color of nobody's skin, flesh-colored shoes which blend in with the rest of the leg must almost always be dyed.

As if you didn't know it, the bride's mother is extremely important to a wedding, and all that goes before it. But, whether at the ceremony itself, or shopping with her daughter for a trousseau, or selecting patterns for china or silver, she should remember that this time her daughter is the star. She should dress in a way to please her daughter, not competitively. Even if the mother is an inveterate jeans-

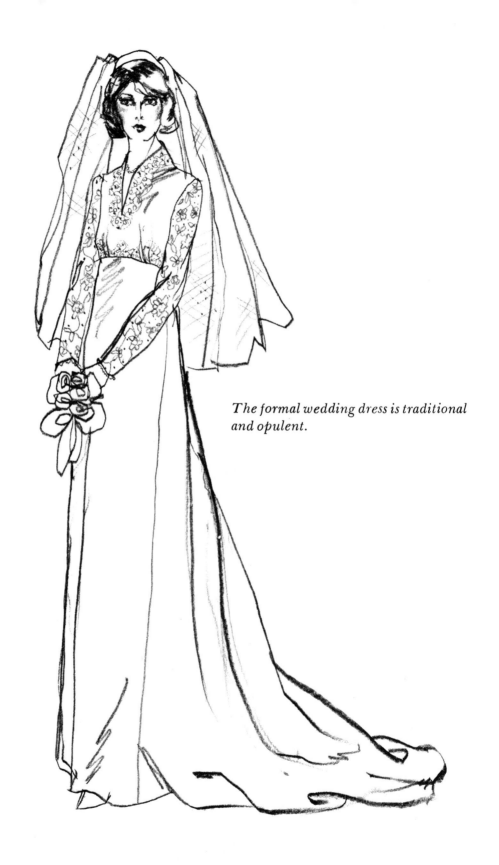

The formal wedding dress is traditional and opulent.

wearer, she should put on a dress, skirt or suit even for the pre-wedding shopping trips. This is an occasion, and the bride's mother should play a supportive, and supporting role, dressing to complement her daughter.

If this is a second wedding (or third, or fourth one), the bride may be the age her mother was when at the bride's first wedding. Then the bride wears light colors, maybe a beige suit or a pale lavender dress. But if she wants to wear white and go the whole first-wedding route all over again, there's no reason why she shouldn't. And if she's middle-aged, that's particularly wonderful. Why shouldn't a woman at forty, forty-five, fifty, fifty-five—whenever—walk down an aisle in a beautiful white dress, on the arm of her son?

If you're going to be a bride, look at your life-style, your personality and his and then decide what kind of feeling you want at your wedding. This is one time when the clothing statement you make can be all fantasy. Perhaps you want to please your parents with an old-style wedding. Or you want to indulge the romantic side of yourself. On the other hand, if you've had the honeymoon before the wedding, if you've been living together for a time and don't want a big fuss made over the wedding, don't be pressured into it. Make your wedding an expression of your dreams. Be a barefoot bride in Central Park or a lacy vision in a church; have eight pastel bridesmaids or two suited witnesses. For once in your life you can more or less write your own script, with you in the starring role.

Dinner with the Boss

MRS. BIG: Will you and your husband join Mr. Big and myself for dinner on the twenty-second?
YOU: We'd love to. . . . (The rest is spoken silently.)

You have to make two major evaluations: the event itself and your wardrobe. First, how formal is it? A large party or an intimate one? At the boss's house or will you be dining out? How well do you know Mr. and Mrs. Big (and all the little Bigs)? Will you be going to a city apartment or a country home? What kind of weather can you expect? When you've resolved these questions, turn to your wardrobe. Don't plan to buy anything special for the occasion unless you absolutely, positively have nothing suitable to wear. And that's unlikely, unless you've spent the past few years in Antarctica.

It's generally not a good idea to rush out and buy something for one particular occasion. You want to wear something you know you'll be comfortable in, that you've worn before and know how to accessorize. A darling watchamacallit that you buy for one occasion is likely to be an extravagance you can't afford.

If It's His Boss . . .

Play a supportive role. Dress with style, certainly, show your creativity and individuality as a dresser, but don't make so strong a statement that you overshadow your husband. This is not your show to steal. Even if you're Joan of Arc to the neighbors, even if your income is higher than his, on this occasion you're coming along as his wife. Go as his partner, not his rival. On the other hand, don't efface yourself to the point where it seems he's brought along part of the furniture.

For an elegant dinner party at their house, choose a simple style in a dressy fabric. The perfect safe outfit would be silk lounging pajamas—or a silk caftan, or a richly embroidered one. The dressy at-home outfit is what's needed, something that shows ease as well as elegance. This would be right for all formal at-home dinners, in city or country, summer or winter.

If the occasion is more intimate, you might choose a long skirt, a flowered challis or a peasant skirt (in satin or bouclé it goes to elegant dinners) with a peasant blouse. Lounging pajamas again are fine, and the material can be less dressy. With pants (satin or velvet), wear a silk or satin blouse, a colorful tunic or overblouse. Or wear a long simple at-home dress.

If it's summer and you'll be dining out of doors, make sure you take a stole. Light cashmere is an excellent choice. In winter, you'll wear a heavier skirt, and if they live in the country, a long tweed skirt with turtleneck sweater and great belt would be a marvelous look.

Remember that almost every outfit you own can be dressed up or down. Unbutton your shirt a little more than you usually do, and add a chain of pearls. Modify the long black dress with a brightly colored scarf tied around the waist or at the neck. Many women buy their at-home outfits in the lingerie section of department stores. Nowadays nightgowns and robes can often serve double duty for bed or dinner. They're of lightweight material, machine washable, easy and flowing on the body and virtually wrinkleproof. They're also a lot less expensive than what you'd find in an evening shop.

The at-home dinner calls for a comfortable, simple look, with legs covered (long skirt or pants). That look covers all occasions from formal to informal, winter and summer, city and country, depending on the fabric and accessories.

If It's Your Boss . . .

And he's not married, I'd recommend you wear the sexiest strapless evening gown you own, with an absolutely divine stole over it. Wear whatever shows you off to the best advantage possible, without over-stepping the bounds of good taste. If it's your boss and he's married, cover up a little more. You should still show off your assets, but don't be obviously competitive. Remember that his wife has a great advantage over you, and that's pillow talk. If you're in your knockout red strapless

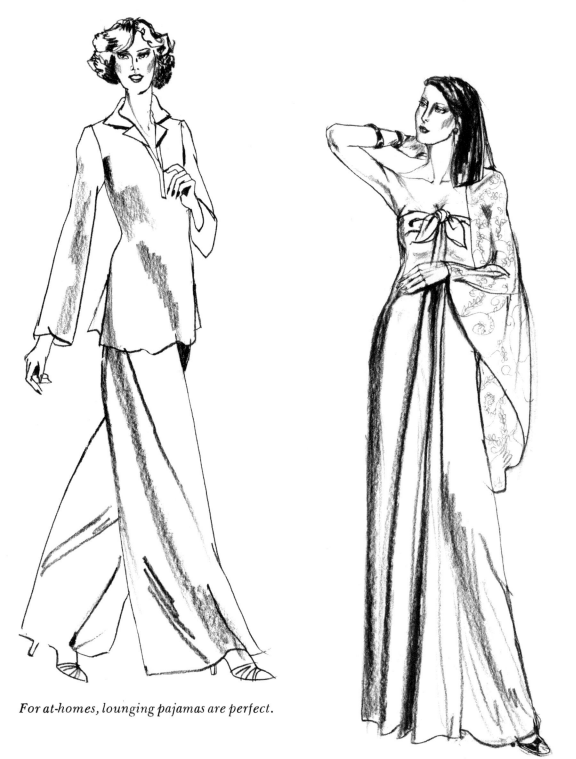

For at-homes, lounging pajamas are perfect.

If you're with your unmarried boss, wear
the sexiest dress you own.

down to the navel, her pillow talk could mean that you'll soon be hunting for another job.

If You're Going Out with the Bigs . . .

Dinner at the race track, or the new French restaurant, or that little Viennese place they've gone to for years all mean a dinner dress.

Every woman needs a dinner dress. In fact, that's one item you can never have too many of. Let me explain: A dinner dress is not a cocktail dress and is not restricted to dinner wear. It's not décolleté, not low-backed, not form-fitting. It has no enormous skirt. It's that perfect simple dress you make interesting by what you do with it. It can be any color. You can wear it to lunch. You get more wear out of it than any other costume you own. It's a dress that crosses all boundaries; it can go to restaurants or private dinners at home, to weddings, funerals, christenings. You could compare a dinner dress to a good steak—simple, understated, fine for lunch or dinner, and with the proper sauces, accompaniments, vintage wine, fare that can be fit for monarchs. So the dinner dress can go from steakhouse to palace by the mere addition of a golden belt, evening shoes and wonderful antique jewelry.

The dinner dress should have a high neck, or a jewel neckline, and can be sleeveless. Short sleeves, cap sleeves, three-quarter or long sleeves are all good. Choose this dress in a light fabric, in the color that looks best on you. Then get another in black or biege or navy or tan. Very few occasions take place after noon where this dress isn't right. It'll go through the day, too: on its own for the little lunch, then garnished with gold or pearls taken out of your handbag for the elegant dinner.

If you're not told what kind of occasion it will be at the Bigs, at least you do know it's at home. Your dinner dress or your at-home outfit (long skirt or dressy pants) are fine. And if you've met the Bigs, it doesn't hurt to ask the hostess, when she extends the invitation, what

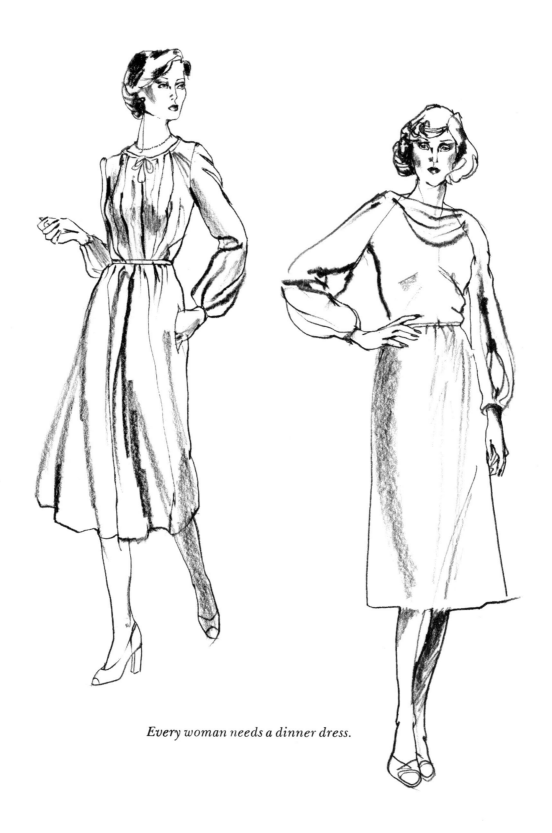

Every woman needs a dinner dress.

she'll be wearing. If she's vague, the dinner is informal. And if it's a barbecue I'm sure you'll leave the satin at home.

Come See the Baby

Come along, everybody, see the pretty
                                    baby,
Such a pretty baby ought to be adored.
Come along, everybody, come and bore
                              the baby,
See the pretty baby, begging to be
                              bored.

—Ogden Nash, *"After the Christening"*

This is the perfect time to take out your wedding outfit again—the one you wore as *guest*, not bride. For a christening, bar mitzvah, first communion, put on that suit or dress. Or wear one a little more extravagant in color—a red or purple knit suit, patterned or plaid or floral. This is a joyous occasion (for everyone but the baby, usually), and with religious significance.

By knit suit I mean something that isn't form-fitting, and not the tailored business suit either. That's too somber. I'm thinking of the Chanel suit—as wonderful an invention as the dinner dress or black velvet pants—that every woman should own, whether it's in a knit, wool, satin or brocade. It's a classic suit that will never go out of style. Even a heavy woman can wear it, though preferably not with a straight or pleated skirt. She'd do better with an A-line skirt, or one that has some give to it.

The dinner dress is also perfect. If it's a christening, and you plan on cuddling the baby, make sure you wear something in a washable

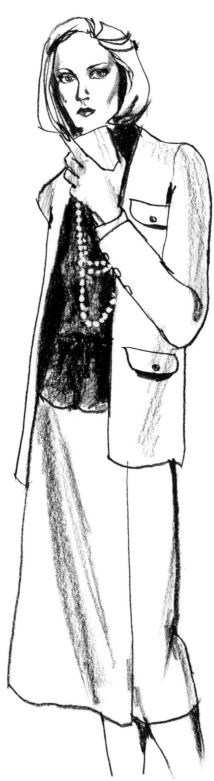

The Chanel suit is timeless.

fabric. Or risk insulting the mother by asking for a towel or diaper to put between you and the little darling.

A boisterous bar mitzvah can be equally dangerous to your clothes, particularly if children and adults are feasting together and the children are not accumstomed to a free flow of wine or champagne (or, even worse, Bloody Marys).

On occasions that welcome a child into life or into responsibility, you dress for the parents. No matter if the child is your favorite niece or nephew, don't dress as though you were going to a children's party. Dress gaily, not cutely. Dress so you're comfortable sitting and standing and dancing. These occasions combine joyfulness with solemnity; let your costume reflect the first in bright colors, the second in simple cut. This is no time to show your bronzed midwinter midriff.

Last Farewell

You're no longer required to wear black to a funeral, but I feel you should always wear dark or "earth" colors—the browns and rusts, no lighter than a café au lait. Deep blue (navy) or forest green are appropriate; so is charcoal gray—and any other deep, somber shade—a "respectful" color.

You don't have to wear a hat, either, unless you are in a Catholic church. It's an option, not a necessity, just as the wearing of black is.

A widow will not consult any fashion guide. She'll probably choose to wear black automatically. Then again, she may not, depending on the husband. (I don't mean depending on whether she liked him or not—though I recently read a book in which the wife wears to his funeral the one outfit she knows her husband hated, as her final statement to him.) I mean that through their intimacy and their relationship, the woman is going to know more than anyone else what her hubsand would have wanted her to wear. She may know that he would not have wanted to see her in black. Maybe he would have wanted to see her in the dress she was wearing when they met, or the dress she was wearing the night he proposed, or his favorite—the outfit he most loved to see on her.

If the widow knows this, or feels it instinctively, she should wear it, and not care what anyone else might think. Even if it's white, or if it's purple—whatever it is. But generally, the widow will feel most appropriately dressed in black, with black stockings and a black hat or veil. The veil is really for her protection, not to make a fashion statement. It's there to protect her from the eyes of people who'll be looking at her, watching her, whether they mean to or not.

The widow will invariably wear what she *feels* is right—and that will always be right.

Guests should be in somber, understated outfits. The last funeral I went to was during the course of a business day. I wore a forest-green cashmere shirtdress by Halston with a dark brown belt and brown boots. I came from the office, carried my briefcase, left it outside and walked in. If the funeral had been on a weekend, when I could have specifically dressed for it, I might have worn something different—though I'd never want to make a fashion statement at such an occasion.

Whether it's a funeral or memorial service, whether the deceased was a good friend, an acquaintance or someone you never knew but admired greatly, it's appropriate to wear anything dark, somber—as long as it isn't "gay." Just think of the word, and look at what you own—any outfit that has "gay" written all over it is something you don't wear. Anything that doesn't have that connotation is acceptable. And beyond acceptability, consider sentiment. If the person who died was close to you, you may choose clothes that represented something to you both.

Dinner at the White House

*The President and Mrs. X
request your presence
at a dinner reception
on the Tenth of November
in the Blue Room
of the White House.*

This is a serious black tie occasion—inky black. It means the most elaborate dressing of all, just one step down from the complete ball gown, which isn't even being designed anymore today. It's the modern version of the ball gown, the most superb thing you own, or, if you don't have it, the most superb thing you're going to own. Though I've advised against running out and buying a special dress for a particular occasion, this is one exception. If you're invited to the White House and don't have a spectacular gown, go out and get one. But don't get something with a neckline so low it looks as though you're planning to get your tan in the Blue Room.

I've been to the White House for state dinners many times and have never worn a gown that would be remotely suggestive. I'm dressed to the teeth, but in a very ladylike way. I think that's imperative. This is not the place to make a strong sexual statement with your clothes.

At an embassy, I will make any statement I wish, though I stay within certain guidelines depending on which embassy it is. I'll dress differently at the Russian embassy, for instance, than I will at the French. At the Russian, I dress down, in something elegant, but without glitter. No sequins or brilliants for the Russian embassy; not too décolleté, either. I choose a more earthy kind of evening gown for the occasion. At the French embassy, I wear *the* most chic, most elegant, most flowing dress I have. I don't worry about the depth of my décolleté—the French

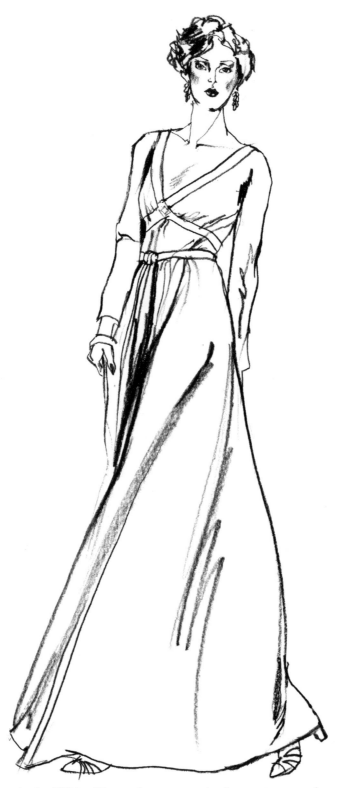

At the White House, be spectacular but not suggestive.

like décolleté. So do the Iranians, and so do all Latins. They love women and love to see them in the most feminine kind of outfits.

At embassies of the East European countries, or at African embassies, I wear rather conservative gowns because I don't want to stand out too obviously amid embassy wives. At Latin or Middle Eastern diplomatic events, I'm much more feminine and female—though never overwhelmingly so. At any Washington affair of this sort, you have to make sure you don't overdo it. I certainly wouldn't wear a cut-out leopard skin, for instance.

If the invitation is for cocktails rather than dinner, you can still wear something long. It may be dressy lounging pajamas, a long skirt or a long understated dress. If you are a national of the country that has invited you, or if your parents were, you might want to go in national dress. If you're not, keep away from it. The national dress then becomes a costume on you and seems patronizing, at best.

When in doubt—at embassies of countries you have little acquaintance with or at nationally mixed United Nations parties—your safest move is always to dress one step down from your original impulse.

For diplomatic luncheons, wear your best-looking suit, your most flattering dressy shirtwaist dress or a liquid, understated dinner dress; just keep away from the tea garden party kind of clothes. You can wear the most vibrant colors—and here's another chance for hat lovers to get good use out of their beloved gear.

In fact, even I once wore a hat to such an event. When I sang at Mamie Eisenhower's birthday luncheon, I wore an electric-blue wool dress—high-necked, long-sleeved—and a marvelous sable-fur hat. It was winter, and one of the few times in my life when I felt I really wanted to wear a hat. (It was also back in the days when hats were worn more frequently. Mamie also had a hat on.)

At other lunches I've worn suits, or dresses with jackets—what I call the costume. This is a perfect occasion for it. But a real "costume" (in the sense of dirndl, dashiki, sari or kimono), though it may be in-

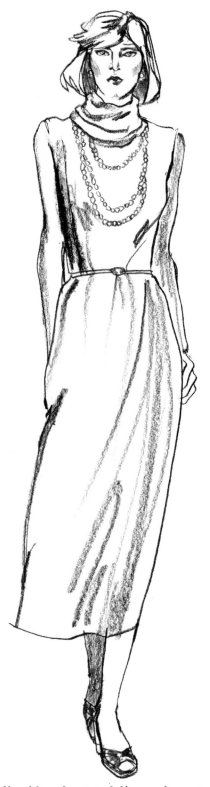

Or wear your liquid understated dinner dress at the White House.

credibly beautiful and you wear it often at home, is totally out of place on such an occasion when it's making a misleading statement about your nationality. Wear clothes that say who you are.

School's Out

Graduation. This is your child's chance to shine. At the same time you know that your child wants to show you off. Every youngster wants to have the best-looking parent there. So you have to tread a narrow tightrope line, particularly if your child is a girl.

Wear something that isn't too outrageous a statement, but is most becoming to you. I've been to a few graduations, including my eldest daughter's graduation from high school, her college graduation and, most recently, to my younger daughter's high school graduation. I find at such times it's wonderful to ask my child what she'd like me to wear.

When a child is graduating from high school, she's certainly reached a time in her life when she knows what she wants to say about herself in terms of fashion. As a matter of fact a child of seventeen or eighteen is much more secure in knowing what to wear than he or she will be ten years later. (At that age you're sure of a lot of things. Doubt often accompanies maturity.)

It's nice to ask your child whether there's any particular outfit you own that she'd like you to wear. If it's something you specifically hate, then, first of all, you can start wondering what it's doing in your closet and, second, you'll still have some idea of the way your child wants you to dress, though you may not wear that particular outfit.

I've worn a costume (dress and jacket) for graduations. For the last one I wore a very simple yellow man-tailored gabardine suit, with a café au lait blouse and a café au lait scarf. I'd worn the scarf as ascot with the blouse, but on this occasion I used it as a sash to dress the skirt up a little bit.

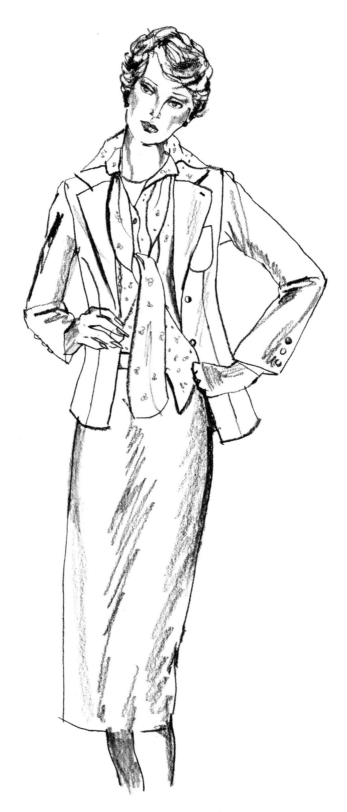

A costume is perfect for graduations.

My graduating daughter wore a long white eyelet dress, high-necked and long-sleeved. Most of the girls wore long dresses, even though the graduation was at eleven-thirty. It's almost as magical for them as wearing a wedding dress—though a very, very, very understated one.

What a girl or woman wears to her college graduation will depend on many things, including how she feels about the event, what kind of college she's graduating from, and what the others are wearing. Generally, she'd wear a dressy, but not formal outfit. It might be white or pastel; it could be a suit or dinner dress. Whether the woman is twenty-one or sixty-five, when she gets her college degree, it's a time to celebrate. She'll wear what makes her feel gay and happy—a celebration outfit.

Class Reunions

Breathless young voice with middle-aged overtones: "Tish, this is our twentieth, you know, and we're all just *dying* to see you, and your husband of course, who we all hear is just *fabulous*, and we'll have . . ."

This time you're going to make a statement to all the people you went to school with about who and where you are now. Or about who and where you want them to *think* you are. It's very important to decide ahead of time what you want to be saying. You may decide that if you let them know how *very* well you've done, several of them may be on you for loans. So perhaps you won't want to make too strong a statement about how successful you've been, or your husband has been.

This is also a time when you'll pick the clothes that make you feel best about yourself, that make you feel very attractive and very comfortable. If you've maintained a great figure, now's the time to let them know it. You can show them you're as young as you were when you graduated. So wear the kind of clothes that show your body, but again, don't be too obvious about it, or they might start speculating that the gorgeous curves aren't really 100 percent you. A well-cut form-fitting dress or suit should do it.

And choose bright colors. Don't look as though you're in mourning for all those passing years. Give a gay and happy appearance. A business suit in the evening is out; unless you want your old chums to think you came for buy-sell transactions.

It's time for laughs and fun, for looking back and looking ahead. It's also a time of scrupulous evaluations. You'll be making your judgments about former classmates, and you can be sure they're making them about you. Look as pretty, relaxed and well-groomed as you possibly can.

Make sure you have a lot of time to get ready. Soak in a bubble bath, give yourself a pedicure. Go through your usual beauty routines in a very relaxed way, pampering yourself. And it's imperative that you go to the hairdresser. (Incidentally, I feel you should go to the hairdresser before any major event. This one is especially important.) However, if you have been waiting for a opportunity to make a change in the way you look, to try something new, this is *not* the time.

Just before a very important moment in your life—whether it's graduation or your first invitation to the White House, your wedding or your class reunion—whatever you do, don't try any major change. It will only make you insecure. You'll feel uncomfortable and nervous because you'll be trying out something you haven't done before. So while there's always the chance that it will work out incredibly well and you'll look fantastic, there's also the very real possibility that you'll hate what's been done, and that will ruin this day or evening that's so important to you.

So go to the hairdresser and have the usual. If you want to try something new, make it your underwear. That way if you love it, you'll glow, and if you hate it, you can assure yourself nobody can see it.

When It's His Reunion

Remember you're traveling as a unit. Again, this is a moment—like your child's graduation—when you're a supporting player, so it's a good idea to ask for advice. Ask your husband what he'd like to see you in, what his favorites are on you.

If you have the kind of husband who says, "Don't bother me with things like that," or "The black one," and he always says "the black one," even though you have ten black outfits or none, then, rather than starting that terrific, predictable fight all over again ("You never notice me"; "Sure I do, I just don't notice what you're wearing"; "You would if you loved me," and so on), you have to do his work for him. Think back to those times when he said he loved you in something and wear that.

He'll need your support now because he's going to be nervous, he's wondering what other people will think of him and the position he's reached and what work he's doing and how well he's done. He'll be nervous about seeing old friends—old buddies and old female friends (who might turn out to look surprisingly well, considering). You should be understanding of his nervousness and at the same time present yourself in a way that will make him proud of you. After all, you are one of his major accomplishments.

The same is true in reverse, of course. He should be supportive of you at your reunion, try to make you as comfortable and happy as you can be. You might not need the support—it could all turn out to be a glorious blast. On the other hand, you might be reluctant to see people who once meant a lot to you and whom you haven't seen for many years. It might not be easy for you to expose yourself to them.

If this is so, and your husband plans to wear something you don't like to see him in, or something you think is inappropriate, then tell him. You don't have to scream, "Omigod, don't wear that terrible suit! Why can't you wear something decent for a change?" You can say, gently, that this occasion means a lot to you and it would please you very much if he'd wear your favorite sports jacket, the one he looks so good in. You don't have to be cute, but I've always found it's more effective to persuade than to command. Some husbands are more insecure about their wife's reunion than their own, so treat him gently.

"Let Me Take You Home to Meet Mother"

Unless he wants you to meet her after your first encounter, chances are you'll know something about him, and her, by the time this invitation comes. You'll have some idea of his background and tastes. The same is true if you're meeting his friends or boss for the first time.

But unless you're completely sure of yourself, or your wardrobe is so limited that there's no possibility of a choice, your best bet is to ask him outright. If you tell him you're a little tense about meeting his parents or friends, and could he advise you on what to wear, you're accomplishing two things at once: He'll be more protective of you, and he'll give you information.

Use your own judgment, too. It's important to wear something that you're very comfortable in. (Comfort is the number-one consideration in dressing for all occasions you're uneasy about. You need all the support you can get, and I don't mean girdles or padded bras.) Feel good about the clothes you choose. You're coping with enough nervousness to begin with; no need taking a chance and trying something for the first time. Again, I would not recommend that you go out and buy a new outfit for the occasion, unless you really and truly hate everything you own. And if that's the case, you're to be congratulated for having landed a new man under those circumstances.

If you've been invited for a family occasion (Thanksgiving, Christmas, a Seder, Mother's Day, a wedding anniversary), make doubly sure you're comfortable and that you like yourself in what you're wearing. For such occasions, it becomes even more important to ask your man what to wear. And if you're taking him home to Mother on her day, or on some other day the family celebrates, include in your invitation a helpful suggestion: "My parents would love to meet you. Will you come for Thanksgiving dinner? It's just family; Dad always wears a sports shirt." Something like that.

In all family get-togethers, the manner of dressing is a matter of family tradition, though it will vary with each family. If your parents wear evening dress for Christmas dinner, don't assume his family will. Maybe theirs is a boisterous affair, with lots of children and grand-children, everyone relaxing in casual clothes. For such occasions you are not trying to make a fashion statement; you want to blend in, join the group. It's similar to finding out, when you stay somewhere overnight, what your host and hostess do about breakfast. In a house-hold where everyone takes the morning meal together, you'd be em-barrassed to be found fixing yourself a cup of coffee before the others. Conversely, if breakfast is everyone's private responsibility, you'd embarrass your hostess by waiting to be served.

So it goes for dressing. Find out what is expected, and then put on an outfit that is both appropriate and makes you feel good.

Guest of Honor

You're about to receive your award, your promotion, your Oscar, your Pulitzer, your gold watch at retirement. All these people have gathered to see you, and no matter who you are, you're scared. You're waiting in the wings or on the podium, with sweaty hands and tingling toes. You clear your throat many times, wondering how that frog got in there. You realize you've lost your voice and that your knees are not strong enough to hold the rest of you up. Every defect you've ever discovered in yourself now vies for the limelight. You curse yourself for having cheated on that diet that promised to make you look thin to the point of emaciation in ten days. You feel the hairs on your head suddenly becoming independent, each going in a different direction. You wonder if the mascara is now under your eyes. Your shoes are too tight (you can't possibly walk anyway) and you forgot your handkerchief, though you know you'll cry when "It" happens.

All eyes are focused on you. This is worse than getting married. You're being introduced by a speaker who has just mispronounced your name. You *knew* it would be awful, and here's the first of many disasters ahead.

It *will* be harrowing. The most you can do for yourself ahead of time is to make sure you're looking as well as you possibly can. If it's a black tie affair, wear the most stunning gown you own, with your favorite jewelry. If it's a luncheon, wear a simple suit or dress. Take your time getting ready. Lay everything out ahead of time—underwear, stockings, shoes (they should be extra comfortable), clothes, belt, scarf, jewelry.

Now turn your attention to your body, skin and face. You will hopefully have gone to the hairdresser, so protect your hair with a cap or scarf. After your bath or shower, use your body lotion or talc, then apply your cologne generously, particlularly in places that might get sweaty (such as wrists, behind the knees, between or under the breasts). Make sure your face is as clean as it can be before you apply your moisturizer.

Take your time. That's most important. If a stocking runs or a nail chips while you're getting ready, you should have the time to remedy the situation.

After you're dressed and made up, look at yourself in a full-length mirror. See if there's anything you can remove from your outfit and still look chic. If there is, remove it. Try sitting down. Are you comfortable? Does anything show that shouldn't? And, perhaps most important, is your skirt wrinkled when you stand up? Definitely avoid

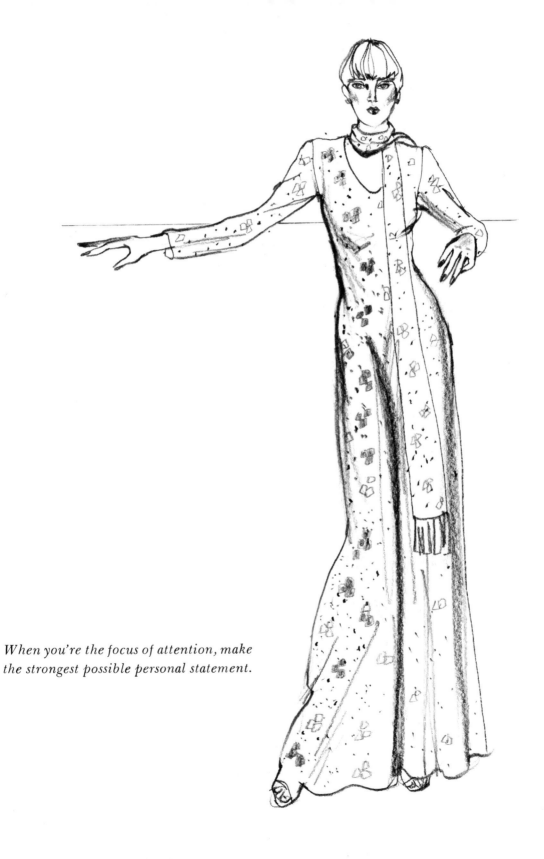

When you're the focus of attention, make the strongest possible personal statement.

that—you don't want to give the impression that you slept in your clothes all night in your eagerness to get the award.

What you're wearing should make the strongest possible personal statement. You are the person being honored for your individual contribution. This is a time to show who you are, not one to dress for possible bachelors in the audience. Wear something that emphasizes your personality, and only subtly advertises your feminine charms.

If you want to buy an outfit or part of one for this occasion, go shopping in plenty of time to make sure you find something you really love on yourself, something that expresses who you are, and that you're comfortable in.

When you're trying it on—in fact, *whenever* you're buying something new—make sure you walk in it and sit in it. I repeat this because I've learned from sad experience. That incredible gown or suit or dress was the most beautiful thing in the world when you were standing in the dressing room. Even walking in it, it was the most graceful, lovely, dynamite thing you'd ever had on in your life. And you walked out in it. Now you go to the dinner. You sit down. You go through dinner, talking and eating. Then you stand up to accept the award. The entire front of the gown looks like an unmade bed.

As you get ready for that award ceremony, remember you'll be watched in all positions—sitting, standing, walking. Pick something to wear that will evoke the same message whatever you're doing, and make that message *strong*.

Auld Lang Syne

For New Year's Eve parties, wear your most swinging outfit, because New Year's Eve is the worst holiday of them all. That's the time when everybody's made up his mind this has got to be the best evening of the year. So automatically, you start out with heavy chances of being disappointed.

Put on your lowest décolleté, the dress or outfit that makes you feel the happiest, gayest, sexiest. And try to leave some of your expectations at home.

Having a Baby

You're pregnant, and you're delighted. Congratulations! But don't rush out to buy an entire wardrobe of maternity clothes in your sixth week. You're going to be pregnant for a long time, and somewhere around the fifth month it may seem you've been (and are going to be) pregnant forever. Then, however thrilled you are to be expecting, you might start to get bored with it all. Some women begin to dislike what's happening to their bodies. They may even hate the way their bodies look. Even if they love the whole idea of having a baby, they'll probably go through a few depressions during those nine months.

Hold off on the maternity clothes for as long as you can. And when the time comes when you absolutely have to, go easy. It's not worth investing large amounts in maternity clothes. Buy a rocking chair instead—a nice old-fashioned one with plump cushions. Or get savings bonds for your child. Even if this is your first child, and you plan on having a large family, don't overdo the shopping. By the time you have your fifth, you might hate the scarlet and purple combination that you now adore.

In the early months, chances are you can wear your regular clothes, particularly sweaters, overblouses, tunics, your nightgowns, robes, caftans of course, and all the loose clothing you own.

Also, borrow from your friends. I know many women who can certainly afford to buy new clothes, but who trade maternity garments among themselves. Do that if possible. It's a nice feeling to have a lot of variety in your clothes at this time, even in what you wear around the house. It prevents becoming bored with your two good maternity pants, say, or your one good wool skirt.

What you definitely must buy for yourself are underclothes. Get the best bra you can find, the one that fits you best. Hopefully, it will be pretty too, in lace or satin. But never choose a pretty bra over a well-fitting one, most particularly when you're pregnant. Your breasts will swell, and may even be painful. Your bra should, first of all, help make you as comfortable as you can be, and then help mold your breasts to the prettiest possible line under your clothes. If you plan on nursing, buy a nursing bra shortly before you're due to deliver. Buy *one* for the hospital; you won't be able to predict with complete accuracy what your breast size will be, so it's best to buy additional bras later.

If you need the support of a maternity girdle—usually toward the end of pregnancy to help alleviate back pain—again, get the best you can find. Treat it as a medical aid, not as a fashion item. It's hard to look attractive if you're uncomfortable or in pain, so make sure it gives the most help.

No matter how little you want to spend on maternity clothes, your first priority are the four essential health aids you may need: bra, girdle, hose and shoes. In late pregnancy, your ankles may begin to swell, perhaps even your feet. Your legs might feel tired. You'll want good walking shoes, probably with a little heel (that helps prevent backache). You'll also probably want support stockings, and you'll need a few pairs because you'll be wearing them all the time.

Don't try to borrow the four essentials; these are necessary personal investments and they're unavoidable, whether you plan to have a dozen children or only one. A few lucky women go through pregnancy with no discomfort whatsoever, but it's best to expect that your pregnancy will be average, with the mild aches or discomforts for which you need support.

The specific maternity clothes you have to buy will depend partly on what you already have in your wardrobe that's loose enough; on the time of year or climate during your late pregnancy; and on your life-style. The best rule is: Invest as little as you can on clothes you won't be able to wear later (maternity pants, skirts); invest more on loose tops, gowns and dresses that you can wear forever.

During pregnancy your skin will probably be glowing. Emphasize it with bright makeup, and keep your hair shiny clean and well groomed. Show your arms and hands to best advantage. You probably won't want to wear anything with too deep a décolleté, but if you're comfortable in a dress with a low back, this is an excellent time to wear one. Low-backed dresses are very sexy and very dressy.

When you're getting ready to buy or borrow, you might keep in mind the following:

Basic Maternity Wardrobe

Nightclothes

It's very important to remain as feminine and lovely as possible during pregnancy. Many women feel more feminine now than at any other time. Have a few gorgeous nightclothes. If you plan to nurse later, choose gowns or pajamas that open down the front. Silk or satin pajamas, cut like lounging pajamas or even man-tailored, are excellent choices. They're sexy, comfortable, elegant and keep you warm. Night-gowns should be loose and flowing. Get something frilly if you don't have it, or a luxurious long satin gown. Buy your robe to go with all your nightgowns or pajamas. Have comfortable slippers. Get a lacy and feminine bed jacket (one or two or three) for the hospital.

Pants

These you will not be able to wear later. Buy no more than two dressy pants and two casual pants or jeans. (But better yet, try to borrow.)

Skirts

Same problem as pants. Get only what you absolutely need for those few months.

Tops

Now you can invest. Tunic tops are marvelous and are always in style, particularly the short caftanlike ones to be worn over pants and skirts. All types of overblouses are good—burnooses and dashikis, ponchos and kimonos. And all of these can be bought in a variety of stores, without ever having to go to a special maternity shop.

Dressy outfits/evening wear

Don't buy that one magnificent expensive outfit. You'll want some variety, even in those few months. Best choices are: dressy caftans, lightweight lounging pajamas, long dinner dresses in a rather heavy crepe or jersey that will fall in a straight line to the ankles or floor. The long dinner dress will take you almost everywhere in the evening, from a black tie event to an at-home dinner where your man may be in a sports jacket or a turtleneck sweater.

I went to a concert at George Plimpton's when his wife Freddy was expecting. She wore a beautiful Jean Muir dinner dress in a very lovely purple crepe that dropped gracefully to the floor. It had a jewel neck and small cap sleeves. I wore a velvet pants suit. The men were either in suits or in Levis and sports jacket. Freddy was neither over-dressed nor underdressed. She looked stunning.

That's the kind of dress I'd consider perfect. You can wear it to anything from six in the evening on, even to the White House. And you can wear it right up to the moment . . .

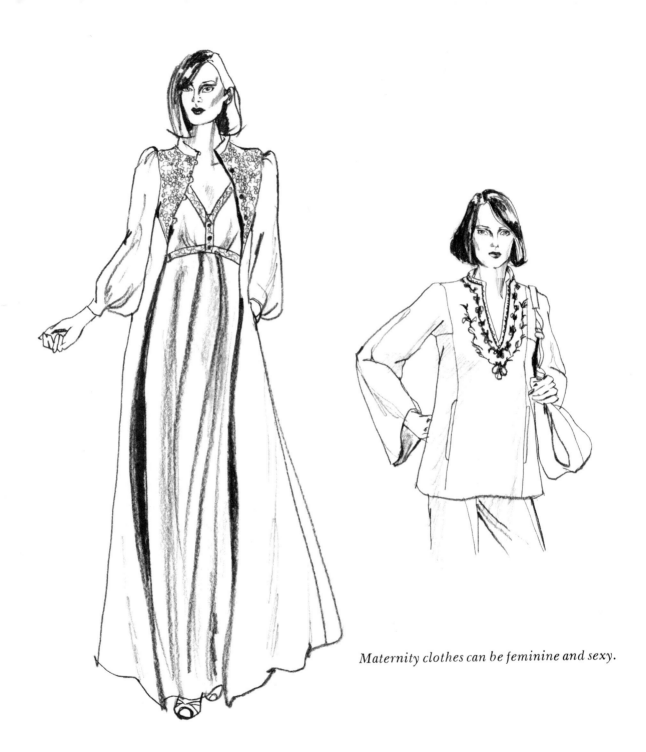

Maternity clothes can be feminine and sexy.

When the baby comes

It's five in the morning and you're in labor. This is not a very good time to start packing a suitcase. Don't wait until the cramps are three minutes apart. Have your suitcase prepacked and ready to go at least ten days before your due date.

Pack your most beautiful bedclothes, gowns and bed jackets. People will be coming to see you and the baby, and they'll expect you to be beautiful and radiant. Pack your robe, even if you have a private room. You might want to stroll down the hall and peek into the nursery. Take comfortable slippers.

Pack toiletries, makeup, moisturizers, scents. It's a good idea to take along hot curlers, so you can do a fast pickup on your hair when you start to receive guests. If you have long hair, put in a few ribbons to tie your hair up prettily.

Pack the book you wanted to finish reading. If it's very heavy going, put in light reading too; you may feel too happy and excited (or exhausted) to concentrate on philosophy. Take your needlework or crocheting, crossword puzzles, portable chess or backgammon (for when you have visitors), cards for playing solitaire, sketch pad—whatever you enjoy doing. Your body will be recovering from the great event, and you may find it hard to sleep at times.

The suitcase you pack for having a baby is basically the same as for any other time you go to the hospital. Pretty bedclothes are always a good idea, to cheer you up.

For coming home, take something loose, a tunic or shirtwaist without fitted waist. You can't predict exactly what size you'll be, and you probably won't be able to fit into your regular clothes just yet. Even if your weight goes down to your prepregnancy norm, your waist will still be large (though you'll feel absolutely skinny). Take something you love for coming home in; you'll be returning with a new person in your arms!

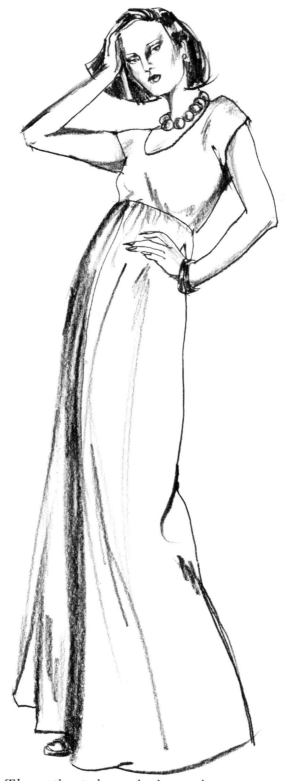

The mother-to-be can look stunning at a party.

For nursing, particularly if you're nursing "on demand," always wear something that's easy to open. Forget your turtlenecks for a while. Stick to cardigans, skirts, and clothes with zippers or buttons down the front. It's not fair to the baby if you come to it hot and bothered because you had to make an elaborate change before feeding. And if you plan to miss a feeding when going out (with someone else at home to give the baby its bottle), make sure you take along nursing pads. Many nursing mothers have been forced to leave a party before they'd planned because their cups runneth over.

3

Dressed for Business

What you're wearing will tell people whether you mean business or monkey business. Clothes, the strongest statement you make about yourself to strangers, announce your status, real or desired. They tell the world: "This is who I am. This is what I do."

It's imperative for the woman in business to dress *positively*. Positive dressing is the nonverbal equivalent of saying, "I'm in charge here." It doesn't mean dressing like a man, or competing with men. It also doesn't mean flaunting your attributes as a woman. It's dressing for the work to be done—announcing that you and it are important.

You can always spot the woman who works and the woman who doesn't work. It's not because high-echelon women look masculine in any way. They're always elegant, with an understated elegance, with casual chic. They're extremely well put-together; a lot of care has gone into their dressing, but you don't notice that. You notice the woman herself. Her clothes provide the background for the individual competent personality. Only when you look closely do you see that everything is just right and well thought out.

The secret of positive dressing lies in two words: comfort and chic.

If a woman has any ambition, she should learn to make a positive statement about herself through clothes. If you are a secretary or typist, and you don't ever want to be anything more than a secretary or typist, then you can afford to dress any way you like.

If, on the other hand, you work in an office and have a desire to get ahead, then you should dress as though you were in charge. There doesn't have to be any difference between the way a woman executive dresses and the way her secretary dresses. The only difference will be in the quality of the fabric. A woman executive can probably afford to spend more on her clothes. Her shirt may be pure silk, while her secretary's is synthetic. But only the minutest inspection will show up these differences. The secretary can be just as chic as her boss. And, chances are, she could become just as successful.

You notice the power of positive dressing immediately. Salespeople, waiters, cab drivers treat you differently. You move up in status, your position is respected. You get a better table in the restaurant, the taxi comes straight to you, the salesperson looks up smartly when you walk in.

The rules for positive dressing are very simple. Even if you want to be the Total Woman at home, if you enjoy wearing little peekaboo knickknacks, you can still command respect and attention during your workday, if you'll follow one simple rule: *When you're in business, dress for business.*

This is not the time or place to make an all-out effort to get a man. You can do that after working hours. What you wear should be saying: I am here for business, at least right now—not, I am here for play.

The style in which you dress announces how you spend your day and what you do for a living. Some women earn their living a certain way, and dress a certain way on street corners to announce their business. It's a form of advertising.

If you work in an office, and you want to look as though you're in charge, the most important thing to remember is *understatement*. Comfort and chic are the two words to hold in mind when you're selecting your business clothes.

When you shop, buy clothes that can live well throughout the business day. If you look great at 9:00 A.M. and withered by lunch hour, you're wearing the wrong things. Choose fabrics that don't wrinkle easily. Synthetics are excellent—easy to care for and not hard on the budget. Those that most closely resemble natural fabrics—wool, cotton, silk—are best.

Choose clothes that hold their shape well. Straight tight skirts are obviously a rotten choice for the office. They're uncomfortable, they ride up and, when you stand, they'll show you've been sitting all day. If straight skirts look good on you, get one with inverted front and back pleats. It gives the look of a straight skirt and still has leeway.

A skirt can be body-revealing, as long as it's not too obvious. It can show you have a terrific fanny as long as it has some flow to the hemline. It can drape well over the upper part of your legs and hips, but it must have some give or freedom to it.

With your skirt, wear a smart sweater, turtle- or V-necked. Put a scarf in the V-neck, or wear a blouse under it, for a soft effect. You *can* show that you have a nice figure and still be totally business-like.

Your best bet in a blouse is a silk or silk-synthetic shirt, man-tailored or slightly more feminine (still basically tailored, though), with perhaps a floppy bow that ties at the neckline. Have a cardigan to go over it, or a great jacket, in wool or velvet. The office can get very cool; even if the outside temperature is a hundred degrees, you'll be inside with the air conditioning.

A sweater set looks very chic with your skirt, particularly if it's the same color. That gives you the long and lean look, which you can emphasize with a long gold necklace or a chain of pearls.

Dresses should be simple: a shirtwaist in either summer or winter fabric, a simple sweater dress with a self-tie belt. Pants suits are okay if they're very chic. A playful outfit is not right for the office, and neither are jeans. There are pants and pants. Make sure you know which are which. Well-cut pants with matching jacket are fine. Don't wear pants that you'd put on for a game of sandlot softball. Pants with jokes on them, with patches or tears are definitely out. Office pants should have a tailored look.

One reason why top restaurants waited so long before they broke the clothes code against women in pants is that most women have a tendency not to recognize the difference between pants you'd wear to the movies and pants appropriate to the office or to a smart luncheon. There's a very definite difference, and if you're not sure you see it, my advice is to leave the pants at home. On the other hand, if you hate yourself in skirts, or feel more comfortable in pants, try a well-tailored gabardine pants suit.

In whatever you're wearing, avoid big prints and clothes that are too colorful. Don't wear anything that's flashy. No shocking pink tights; no long, dangling earrings; no jangling bracelets. If you like a print, choose one that's small and unobtrusive. Tweeds are fine, and so is a salt-and-pepper fabric.

Black, on the whole, is not very practical for the office. Obviously it will pick up lint, hair, small bits of paper and anything else that's around. If you do choose black, make sure you carry a tape delinter and be prepared to spend a preposterous amount of your time dealing with your problem. Perhaps this is my prejudice. Some women seem able to wear black and keep it immaculate.

Geraldine Stutz, for example, president of Henri Bendel, is a very individualistic, stylish female executive who always dresses superbly and makes a very strong personal statement. Gerry wears a lot of black, particularly black knit skirts in cashmere or wool, with a wonderful, eccentric hemline (midcalf) that I love. She'll wear a matching cashmere sweater set, dark stockings and shoes to match. I've never asked her how she keeps the black absolutely clean. I can only guess that she spends a lot of time delinting; or more likely, someone follows her around all the time, cleaning her outfit.

However, she does it, she looks sensational. She'll always have one strong focal point—either a beautiful necklace, a great pin placed strategically on the shoulder, a stunning gold belt, or a brightly colored scarf, that she wears wound or braided as a belt. She very rarely wears pants, but often wears a turban.

Gerry's look is very long and lean. She almost never wears two different colors (except for an occasional highlight of color through a scarf). She also happens to be long and lean, but for those of us who aren't, the solid-color way of dressing is the simplest for achieving that look.

It may take a little while to develop a strong individual fashion statement. But American women have the advantage of the finest classic daytime sportswear in the world. That means uncluttered lines, no fuss, easy sophistication. With all the designers creating this style, it's almost impossible to go wrong. Simple chic and casual elegance are their hallmark, and also that of the successful woman.

When you shop, think of how you'll mix and match your clothes later; otherwise you'll have the unnecessary expenses of a very large wardrobe. Buy skirts and tops that can be changed around to create three or four times as many looks. You complete the outfit by wearing your wool or velvet jacket.

Remember: Positive dressing means you look as though you're in charge. You're in charge of your clothes, too. You have made them a backdrop for your *self:* People notice you first; only secondly do they see that you've put yourself together in a very chic, simple way. You're well-groomed too; everything about you is in place.

To summarize, dressing for business means:

1. Understatement.
I can spot the powerful women in a restaurant because they are much

more underdressed than the women who are lunching with girlfriends or with a male friend. The nonworking woman is dressed more "frivolously." I don't mean that in a derogatory way. It's just that she's dressed more obviously like a *female*. Her clothes are softer and more elaborate. She has on more jewelry, and her clothes are more colorful. She's more apt to be in a print than the businesswoman.

2. Casual elegance.

The clothes you wear should be able to take you from the office to a board of directors meeting to perhaps a romantic luncheon (just remove the ascot, or tie your scarf lower, or add jewelry). One small change can usually give a softer, more "feminine" look. The outfit looks fresh at all times. No wrinkles, dust or stains.

3. Good quality.

Buy the best quality you can afford. It's always a good investment. Most women executives I know buy clothes that aren't seasonal; they have a single-season wardrobe of thin gabardines, light wool—the different light fabrics (natural or synthetic) that can be worn throughout the year.

4. Maximum chic without the put-together look.

"Interior decorator" dressing is definitely not for business. By that I mean shoes dyed to match a dress, or a dyed-to-match handbag, or a cute little hat. Your total look should give the impression of naturalness, even spontaneity. Spend hours planning and selecting your wardrobe, but don't let a minute of it show!

5. Neatness.

Whatever you do, if you're going to be out all day, *always* carry an extra pair of stockings (or panty hose) ln your bag. I'm never without it. It doesn't matter if you're in the most elegant Halston; if you have a run in your stockings, a spot on your blouse or a button missing, you are not dressed for business.

6. Minimal jewelry.

Your jewelry, like your clothes, should be understated. A single or double strand of pearls is fine. A gold chain is elegant; it can be either thin and plain or with a medallion, a Maltese cross or an animal— anything that's not too elaborate or obtrusive. Earrings should be simple: small pearl, gold or silver. A hoop earring is acceptable if the hoop is really small. Drop earrings, swinging earrings and large hoops are not right for the office. If you look good in large earrings, take them along in your bag to wear for cocktails or dinner after work. But large, dangling earrings are almost never suitable for daytime wear— except when the occasion is a party or something equally lighthearted. No clanking bracelets either. Wear a simple watch or form-fitting bracelets. You can wear two or three different ones, as long as they don't move on your arm or wrist. There's nothing more disconcerting at a business meeting than jangling or clanking jewelry.

7. Less is more.

The business woman wears nothing elaborate or fussy. No frills or ruffles; no elaborate hairstyles; no excessive makeup. Shoes should be elegant, sensible and comfortable; outrageous heels are out. Bags and briefcases should be efficient. If you carry a briefcase, let your handbag have shoulder straps, to free one hand. A workingwoman's bag should be roomy enough to carry whatever she needs without cramming. It should also be organized. If a woman has to take everything out of her bag to find the one item she's looking for, she gives an immediate impression of being disorganized in her work as well.

Dressing for business means making the best possible impression, and feeling good while doing so. It doesn't mean forgetting you're a woman —but, equally, it doesn't mean stressing the fact that you are one. No- body will make a mistake about your sex. But they might make a mistake about your intentions if you dress for a party when you're at your job. You can dress to show your attractiveness and your authority at the same time if your motto for dressing is: comfort and chic.

The Business Bag

A woman's handbag is traditionally very private. Even a woman's lover knows that her bag is her own affair. Psychological reasons are sometimes given for this, but whether they're true or not isn't our business here. A woman's purse is also part of her working equipment, as is her briefcase, so bags and baggage deserve the same serious attention as the rest of a businesswoman's wardrobe. I have to carry both every day of my working life, so here's a special note on bags and baggage.

Invest in a good handbag. A cheap one will end up costing you more than an expensive one, since you'll have to replace it after a few months. Two good leather handbags are all you need—one in black, the other in tan, or deep café au lait. The bag should be attractive, of course, but mainly it should be practical. If it's too small, it's useless. And if it's a big donkey bag, you'll never find anything in it.

Think of what you'll be carrying daily. You'll probably need room for many of these items:

Wallet, credit card holder, comb and brush, atomizer, stockings, makeup bag, handkerchief or pocket tissues, cigarettes and lighter or matches, eyeglasses or sunglasses in holder, rain bonnet, extra jewelry, scarf, notebook, pens, appointment book, phone book, keys.

You must have a place for everything, and a bag that comes with compartments will help you organize. As I've said, a disorganized bag reflects on its owner.

A makeup bag within the handbag allows you to keep all the makeup you need in one place. When you go for a touch-up after work, or before lunch, you can do it quickly and easily with everything together. This saves you time and helps keep your bag uncluttered. Even when bags have special compartments for makeup, I prefer a separate makeup bag.

I always carry a notebook with me. In addition, I have a combined appointment book–address book. Here, I keep a short list of phone numbers and addresses (both business and personal) I'm most likely to need. Though I keep a master phone book at home, and another one in the office, the one in my purse assures me that I'll always have essential numbers at hand.

Since I have to carry a briefcase every day, I choose a shoulder bag. This gives me more freedom—to hold a newspaper, umbrella or whatever else I might want to carry.

When you buy your briefcase, think of how much it weighs empty. Don't buy that beautiful, impressive one with the heavy frame. The work you'll have to carry will be heavy enough without lugging extra weight. A soft briefcase is practical and attractive—just make sure it has handles. The kind you carry under your arm may be pretty, but it's not practical.

Think of your handbag and briefcase (or portfolio) as serious, professional equipment. Avoid anything that soils easily or requires a lot of care. And don't waste your money on something that doesn't give you the room you need and creates a frivolous impression. When a woman carries a little bag, you know right away she's not into anything serious.

The Job Interview

Dress for the job you're hoping to get. If you're applying for the lead in a porno film, wear something that shows off your figure and comes off easily. If it's for a modeling job, reveal your figure in a different way, in clothes that move easily and drape well over your body.

Whatever the job, act and dress the part. A first impression is always important, but in this situation it may be the only impression. Your appearance will be making a statement to your prospective employer, and this time the statement you make should be part of a script.

In other words, you'll be acting. Your clothes statement may not be

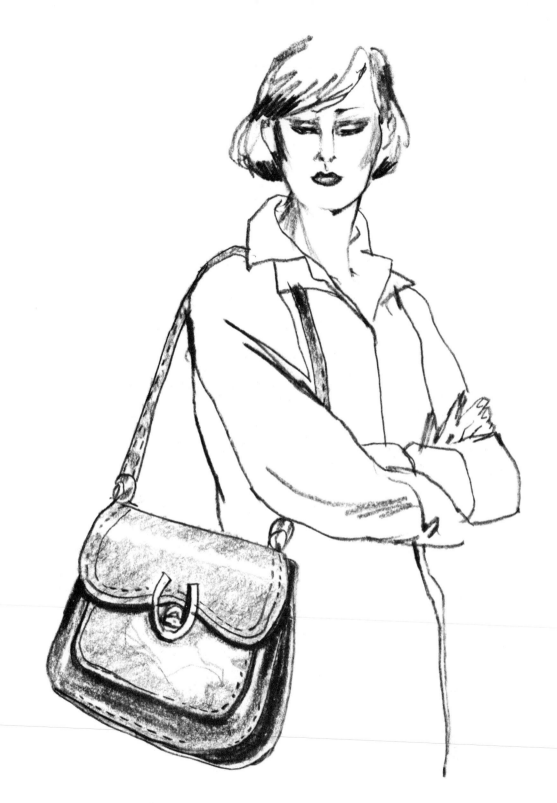

Choose a handbag with room for everything you need.

about the real you so much as about your qualifications. If you're hunting for an office job, don't wear a man-hunting outfit. The best it can get you is a dinner invitation from the interviewer. If you want to catch a man, fine. If you want to land the job, no. For a no-nonsense business job, you wear a no-nonsense business outfit.

That's something all actresses must learn, and it's the first thing a budding actress is taught. When you're trying out for a part, you dress for that part. Most people, even casting directors, are very shortsighted and will not see you as anything other than what's consistent with your appearance.

If you're trying out for a sexy, vampish kind of role and you're wearing a Grace Kelly kind of suit, with short white kid gloves and a pearl necklace, chances are you won't get the part—even if you're perfect for it. Or the reverse: If you're trying out for a ladylike role, and you wear a low-cut blouse, very tight skirt, tottering heels and a lot of makeup, chances are they won't see how right you could look in a ladylike business suit. Wear the sexy outfit when you're trying out for the prostitute-with-a-heart-as-wide-as-all-outdoors role and bring back the little pearl necklace for the Grace Kelly part.

Because most people won't see beyond your appearance, and will take you for what you seem, the most important statement you can make at an interview is made with your clothes. If you're about to be interviewed for office work, don't wear an outfit designed for curling up on the boss's lap. The boss may be a woman, or a man who believes business should remain business. On the other hand, don't forget you're a woman, either.

Let the way you present yourself show that you're a woman. Many women make the mistake of thinking that if they are going into business—into an area run mainly by men—that they must compete with the men on the same level. So they wear a business suit, common-sense heels, and come on with a very businesslike, aggressive, almost macho attitude.

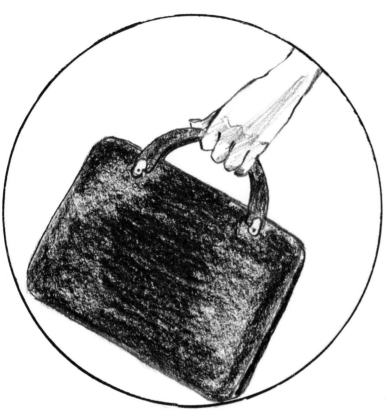

A briefcase doesn't have to look masculine.

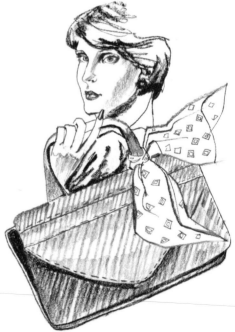

I don't feel that's the right approach. I'm a businesswoman, and that's the way I think of myself. I also think of myself very specifically as a woman, and I make no effort to appear anything other than that.

Whatever you hope to do with the job later, your first consideration is getting it. You won't have a chance to meet the boss who is single and attractive if you don't get the job in the first place. If you go in for the job interview looking both businesslike and as attractive as you can, your chances will be strong.

From then on—unless you want to be known as a business brain who is mainly out to get the boss—you have to be very careful about the way you dress. I don't believe in the old tight-sweater–tight-skirt routine at work, no matter how determined you are to get the boss.

You can wear a suit that's soft and feminine-looking. There are too many obvious women around the office. Why don't you try competing on a different level? The boss will probably notice you sooner, and you'll avoid the antagonism of your female co-workers.

If you're applying for a sales or service job, it will make some difference whether your customers are men or women. If you'll be mainly selling to (or taking orders from) men, wear something that makes you look attractive and feminine, but is also very comfortable and easy to move around in. If you'll be dealing mostly with women, it's very important to dress noncompetitively.

Women will latch on to the competitiveness and be turned off by it. They won't trust you. If you'll be selling clothes to women, don't try to conform to some particular "well-dressed" image. Each customer will have a different idea of what being well-dressed means. The safest route is to wear a basic dress or skirt and blouse. If it fits you well, is the right color for you, you may look stunning. But it'll still be under-dressed, not competitive.

If you have a suit that's really comfortable, you might wear it. But, generally, a suit can be constricting when you're helping a woman in

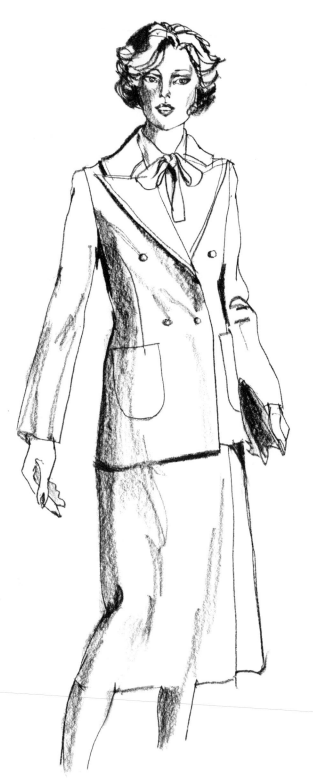

Aim for a suit that's both businesslike and attractive.

and out of her clothes, carrying things or taking orders. A waitress, too, will probably find that it gets in her way. If your job requires that you're physically active, make sure your clothes give you the body freedom you need to get the job done.

Some of these suggestions apply more to the job itself than to the interview. But if you dress as though you're already on the job, your chances are very good that you soon will be.

Working in the Community: School and Civic Affairs

Here again, a noncompetitive attitude to dressing will be most effective. If you wear something to turn on the guys, you'll offend the women, and that's something you can't afford to do. If you're addressing the P.T.A., for instance, you'll be reaching out for the confidence and encouragement of the women—otherwise, you'll never get your plans through. Think of the men in the audience not as handsome guys, but as husbands.

Whenever you're working with women, avoid competition as much as you can. Women sense competition. Nothing will turn a woman off to another woman faster than feeling that woman is competing with her. This is true whether you're working with women or for them, whether they're your employees or customers. In community affairs, particularly, avoid competition in the way you dress. If you're not issuing challenges to a duel, don't dress as if you were.

You don't want to be dowdy either. Women generally notice what you wear more than men do. Men will notice the general effect more than a particular article of clothing. Even if he's lived with a woman for years, a man might not know what's in her wardrobe. That's why some husbands will only offer "the black thing" when asked what to wear, and others will say "don't bother me," or "I don't know." They might be embarrassed not to know; even if they've paid for the article themselves, they might not remember it until they see it again. And they might not recognize it on still another occasion, if the accessories are unfamiliar.

Women are much more observant. It has to be a woman who tells you, "I've *always* loved that dress on you." Women notice the color, cut, stylishness of an outfit, and all the details that put it together into a look. To avoid competition you don't have to be a schlump. Dress attractively. If you want to dress in a strongly individualistic way, or in very stylish clothes, go ahead. As long as you're not being competitive. Signs of competitiveness are a dress that's too tight, a top that's too low, a skirt that's hugging you for dear life.

Wear brilliant colors if they suit you, or the latest style of jumpsuit, but don't wear anything that's too clinging or too revealing. The basics are always safest. You can't go wrong wearing basic business clothes to all civic affairs. The shirtwaist dress, gabardine suit, tailored blouse, well-cut skirt will always give the impression that you're serious about what you're doing, and in control.

If you want people to know you're not taking the situation seriously, or that you'd much rather be someplace else, wear jeans or work clothes. For all but the most casual occasions, such an outfit signals the message that you don't want to be responsible. Even if you're meeting your child's grade-school teacher for a fifteen-minute conference, don't come in jeans. Presumably these fifteen minutes are important to you. Show her that they are.

Jeans belong to a totally relaxed situation; they announce that you want to be comfortable and want to have fun. The minute you wear them to any kind of meeting, you're creating a frivolous appearance which will detract from the seriousness of the event and your ability to contribute to whatever is (or should be) happening.

There is an exception, though: If you're wearing a very chic, tailored jeans suit, you're no longer in the "play" category. There are jeans suits that can take you to luncheons, and such a suit would certainly be appropriate for school meetings and other community events. But knockabout, dragabout clothes shouldn't be worn unless you're knocking about.

With overalls and jumpsuits, again there's a fine distinction. You'll have to judge for yourself if the material, style and cut can carry the statement, "This is important to me." Some women look sensational in jumpsuits, but there's always the bathroom factor. You have to be prepared to do a complete strip. It makes going to the bathroom an event, and you keep putting it off and putting it off until the posssibility of choice is taken away from you. I wouldn't recommend it for women with cystitis or any kind of bladder ailment. A jumpsuit may look beautiful on, but before you buy it, think of how many times a day it will have to come off. And before you tie the belt or scarf around it, remember this is one time when an accessory has to give access.

Working in the community should not be very different from working in an office. You will still be identifying yourself and conveying the importance of what you're doing. Others will respect you more if you dress with (and for) authority. In school events, your appearance reflects on your child, and the importance you attach to his schooling. If you're in charge, or if you want people to think you're in charge, dress positively.

Working in Politics

If you're running for local office, working with the League of Women Voters, with a party or for a candidate, be guided in your wardrobe by "importance" and "noncompetitiveness." What you're doing must be important or, presumably, you wouldn't be doing it. Say that with your appearance. If you're not campaigning for a return to the range, don't wear jeans (again, with the exception of an elegant jeans pants

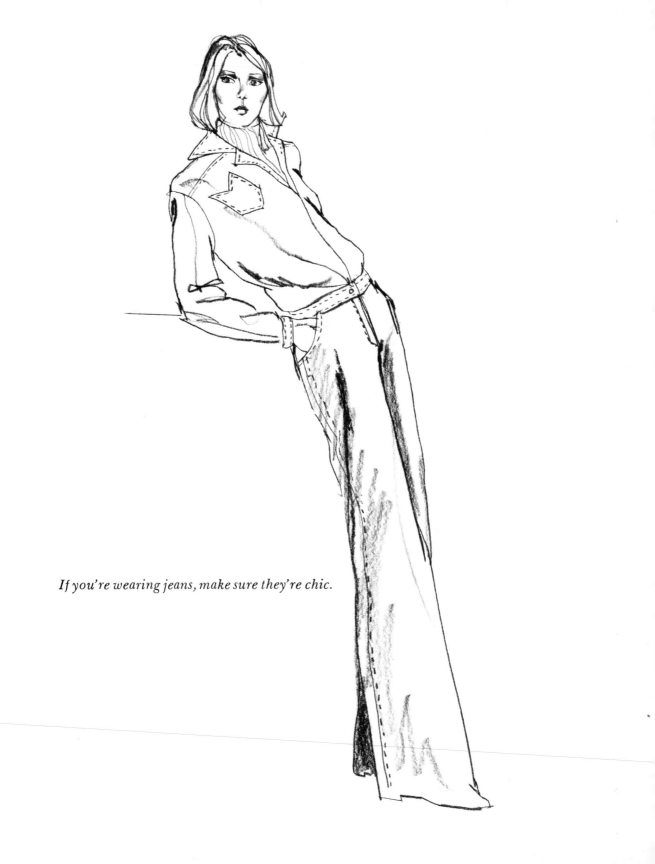

If you're wearing jeans, make sure they're chic.

suit). If you wear clinging clothes, the women in your community might cling to your opponent.

You're in a selling position. You want to inspire trust. You want people to believe that what you have to sell is important and valuable —and that *you* are important and valuable also. Whether you're in an office or canvassing, give yourself the advantage of inspiring confidence on the first impression. If you're going door to door, be even more understated than you'd be in the office, so that if someone answers the door in a dressing gown or painter's clothes, she or he won't have the sense of being "shown up." Anyone who comes to an office will be dressed for going out, but people at home are not necessarily expecting visitors, and it's good business (or politics) to avoid making those you're trying to convince feel embarrassed or insecure in any way.

You know your community, and by looking at its leaders you have a clue as to what style of dressing is trusted. If you live in a very informal area, pants might be appropriate, as long as they're well-fitting and discreet. No matter how informal your neighbors are, don't come to their door in baggy trousers or in pants so tight that the first impression is you're selling something a lot more personal than a candidate or issue. A pants suit allows you to be informal and businesslike at the same time, and will give a more capable impression than pants alone.

If you sense that some people in the community have a bias for women in skirts, wear skirts. Whatever statement you're making about yourself now should be tuned in to what you're selling. Your clothes should not be saying, "Look at me!", but rather, "Listen to what I have to tell you." You are important, yes—but to the cause or person you're working for. Even if you are running for office, you won't get a chance to explain your position if you elicit a negative response at the door. You want people to hear you, and it's very important not to stop their ears through their eyes.

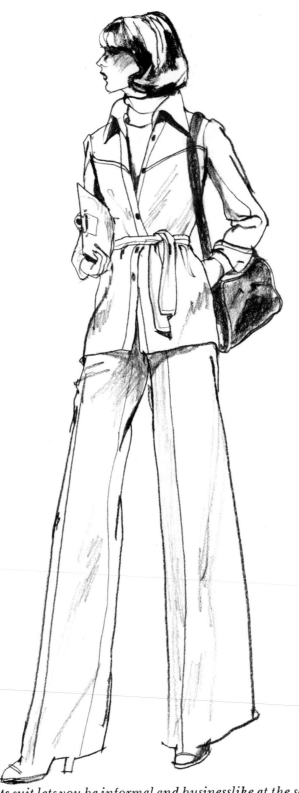

The pants suit lets you be informal and businesslike at the same time.

Dressed for Business

People will take you as seriously as you present yourself. You're selling and advertising your cause. The self-respect you display will reflect on what you have to say. Make sure you look neat and well-groomed. If you hair needs washing, cover it with an attractive turban or scarf. Remember to always carry an extra pair of stockings. If your appearance shows neglect, you will not be taken seriously.

When you're in politics, you mean business. Make that statement in what you wear.

Working in Institutions

People who live in institutions are probably more sensitive to clothes than anyone else. Whether in hospitals, sanitariums, nursing homes or prisons, inmates and patients lead a monotonous existence; almost everything in their life is regulated (including clothes, often) and there's little variety, individuality or spontaneity. A visitor is an event. Anyone who comes in from the outside is the subject of curiosity and interest, even if that person comes in every day as a worker or volunteer.

If you work in (or visit) an institution, remember that you'll be bringing in a lot of information about the outside world. You're telling inmates about life in the big world and on the streets. The women especially, but also the men to a large extent, will be interested in finding out what the fashion is, what women are wearing nowadays. If it's an all-male institution, the men will be inspecting you far more closely than usual, in an effort to read a message about women and their present life-style. Older people will be looking for a message about the younger generation.

Be as attractive and as contemporary as you can without being competitive or aggressive. People who are incarcerated are more vulnerable than others. Be sure to avoid anything too blatant or strident in your appearance or people will shrink from you. They want to learn, not be overpowered.

Wear the brightest colors you own, though. Most institutions are drab, and most people seem to crave color. Remember the pleasure you felt in *The Wizard of Oz* when, after a black-and-white beginning, Dorothy steps into a land of gorgeous color? Color is joyful and hopeful and can almost be a gift in itself when brought into institutions. Wear the happiest colors you own; put on the most upbeat colors and attitudes in dressing that you have.

While you'll want to look as pretty as you can—particularly in male institutions—don't try to be provocative. That's unfair and in doubtful taste. The men want to see the prettiest woman possible—often they're not seeing any women at all—but they really don't need titillation. It's a cruel way of building up your own ego if you're coming on as available in front of those for whom it's of no avail.

Wear feminine clothes. It's uplifting for the patient or inmate to see feminine prettiness. A skirt or dress is preferable to pants in a place where most people are in pants. Also, it shows your legs, and even a little bit of leg goes a long way for people who're not used to seeing them.

Your grooming is especially important. Your appearance should be neat, your hair well done, your makeup well applied. You're bringing in health as much as information, and though you don't want to flaunt it (no total-body instant tan, for example), you do want to bring a sense of well-being into the institution.

You'll want to show visible health and a sense of some gaiety, but without appearing too privileged. The people you are visiting are definitely disadvantaged, whether they're flat on their backs in hospital beds or trapped in an army camp, prison or nursing home. Your freedom is an obvious fact, and though you couldn't deny it if you wanted to, there's also no reason to throw it in the faces of those who are incarcerated.

Be guided by how you would like visitors to look when you're sick at home or in a hospital bed. When you go to an institution, or in any volunteer work you're doing among people who are disadvantaged in some way, look as bright, warm, open and feminine as you can without conveying any obvious sexual message. See-through blouses, deep décolletés or body-clinging clothes are tactless and tasteless. You're here to cheer people up, not to frustrate them.

Ready for the Camera

When you're being snapped or shot, go easy. In a photograph, only the frame of your dress comes across. The drape is usually lost. To get an idea of how you'll look in the photo, go to the mirror and squint your eyes. What you'll see is basically the frame of your outfit, and that's generally what will be picked up.

Wear something flowing, with the simplest possible line. Any stiff or uncomfortable fabric will make you sit in an uncomfortable way— stiff and erect, very straight-backed—and you will appear tense or tight in the photo. You'll want your body to appear loose and natural, so choose clothes with an easy, natural line.

If you're wearing jewelry, stay with small items, particularly near the face. Large or chunky pieces of jewelry will distract.

For television appearances, don't forget the color camera. The first time I was on color television I wore a black and white outfit. Choosing two colors against a lot of color was an obvious ploy. I wanted to go against what everyone else would be doing and stand out through understatement.

Also, I wanted people to look at my face more than at my clothes. The black and white meant more emphasis on my eyes, hair and skin tone. This is what I wanted: People would be seeing *me*, my face, and not my costume.

That was the first time. I'll still wear black and white on color television, but I wear other colors too, though never very bright ones.

A deep burgundy yes, but not a bright red, purple or any shocking color. I'm not so much concerned about whether the color will create a glare as I am in having my clothes be a backdrop. If I choose a very bright color, it would be stronger than I am. I want what comes across to be *me*.

It's like wearing very bright eye shadow. People will see the shadow and not the eyes. To best show off your eyes, wear shadow that emphasizes them, brings out the color but doesn't overwhelm them. If you want your face to be noticed primarily, don't draw attention away from it with brilliant colors further down.

Some television performers can make a strong fashion statement and create a reputation around their outstanding way of dressing. Cher is certainly one of these personalities, and it works for her. She's a very exotic-looking woman, with olive skin, black hair and dark eyes. She can carry strong colors without being overpowered by them.

But if you're like me, who has strong contrast in coloring (fair skin, blue eyes), then very bright colors will tend to wash you out.

When you're going in front of the camera, whether for a still photograph or on television, decide what aspect of yourself you want most to come across. Then play up to it or down from it. People will see what you want them to see and the camera will heighten whatever effect you've decided to convey.

Women at Work: Uniforms

If the work you do requires that you wear a uniform, you're lucky. You're not faced with the problem of what to wear every day. You don't have to invest much money in your working wardrobe, and when other women are buying their fifth skirt for the office, you can be out getting a crazy cellophane sarong for after-hours.

Uniforms can be incredibly attractive (look at them on men!), *if* they fit well, are neat and clean and crisp. On the other hand, there is nothing worse than an ill-fitting uniform. It's worse than any ill-fitting costume of your own.

Whatever uniform you wear—as nurse, stewardess, hostess, waitress, doctor, lab technician, whatever—it can be the most stunning outfit you own if it fits as though it's custom-made. Make sure of the fit and see that the hemline is right for you. You'll need more than one uniform to insure that it's always bright and crisp.

Today there are a lot of wonderful new styles in uniforms; there's no reason for a woman to be stuck with a dull, ugly uniform anymore. If you're a nurse or waitress, you have a lot of choice among outfits with pants or skirts, or you can select a dress in any number of styles to best complement your figure. Even when the uniform is totally regulation, as in the armed services, you can look as chic as any fashion model if you'll spend a little time with needle and thread. Can't sew? Take it to a tailor or dressmaker. The cost won't be enormous and you can be absolutely sure it will pay off. If you're wearing the same outfit every day, then you above all women must feel good in it. And you'll find that the better you feel about your uniform, the better you'll feel about your job.

Tailoring your uniform to fit you as perfectly as possible will let you achieve individuality even if everyone else is dressed in exactly the same way. Your figure, your bearing, your face will come across strongly. And your neat appearance will make people think you're the one in charge.

Whatever kind of work you do—at home, in the community, at a desk or in the skies—people will judge you by your appearance. The kind of work you do will naturally influence what clothes you wear. If you're a house painter, I suggest you do not wear your Halston, even if you're painting the White House. If you're chairing the P.T.A.

The Business Look

Right "I'm in Charge Here"	**Wrong** "Don't Ask Me—I'm Not Responsible"
CLOTHES	
simple line	cluttered; confused
same or blending colors	colors at war
smooth, clean, crisp	wrinkles, runs, lint
well-fitting (tailored or loosely revealing)	tight, form-fitting, body-hugging, baggy
plain colors or small patterns	large patterns, loud colors, much contrast
coordinated outfits (suits, dress with jacket, skirt/pants with top and jacket)	noncoordinated outfits
city clothes	country, beach or farm clothes (jeans)
ACCESSORIES	
minimal jewelry: small earrings, fitted bracelets, single chain	elaborate jewelry; jangles, bangles, dangles; large or long earrings, clanking jewelry
shoes: dark or matching color of legs	shoes: bright or contrasting with color of legs; dyed to match dress
headwear: unfussy turbans, scarves	headwear: large or fussy; "cute" hats
handbag: leather, roomy, dark or earth colors	handbag: tiny or fussy, dyed to match shoes or dress; novelty bags
briefcase: professional, leather, with handle (preferably not heavy)	briefcase: anything not professional in material, color or shape

GROOMING

simple hair style; hair neat and clean	elaborate hair style; unkempt hair
well-applied daytime makeup, not obvious	heavy or dramatic makeup
generally well-groomed (nails, skin, hands, etc.)	not well-groomed

don't come in your Linda Lovelace special, and if you're hoping to get a job as Linda Lovelace's stand-in, don't wear a black gabardine business suit.

But beyond appropriateness, there's an important code to dressing. It's very easy to learn and will provide you with status. If you want people to think you matter, dress as though you matter. And that simply means being comfortable *in* and *about* your clothes. You will be comfortable *in* them if they're neither too tight nor baggy—if they stay in place, don't wrinkle too much and are clean. You will feel comfortable *about* them if you know they are chic. I hope that the concept of chic comes across to you in this book. It can include a variety of factors, but the primary one is simplicity. You can never go wrong if your clothes are understated. In all working situations—and in most other situations as well—the best, the most effective, clothes are those that provide a backdrop for the person you are presenting: yourself, or whatever aspect of self you want others to see.

When you're getting dressed, ask yourself these questions about the outfit: Is it comfortable? Is it chic? Is it apppropriate?

If you can answer "yes" to all three questions, you're sure to be in business.

4

Up to Mischief

—Voulez-vous coucher avec moi ce soir?
—Je voudrais bien, mais que vais-je porter?

When you're planning a seduction, make sure you have made all the necessary preparations. They'll depend a lot on who's coming for dinner. Candlelight might make him squint, incense might make him sneeze, perfume sprayed all over the room might put him to sleep. Use your discretion in all the little "effects"; go easy at the beginning and you'll be able to carry out more advanced experiments later on. A glowing fire in the fireplace is certain to be cozy and soothing in winter, but make sure the flue's open or you'll both be smoked out.

If you're wining and dining him, prepare the meal well ahead of time. Even if you think he's looking for domesticity, he hasn't come over to watch you slave in a kitchen. It'll ruin your hair and makeup, and he won't know whether to help you or sit by himself reading your old magazines. For summer seductions, you can serve beautifully garnished cold meals with a bottle of chilled dry or slightly fruity white wine. In winter, prepare something that can be simmering on the stove, or that just needs a moment's attention, like steak or chops.

Fondues (either cheese or meat) are wonderfully romantic meals, letting the two of you dip and chat and linger.

Buy reliable wines, and if you don't know about wine, ask for advice. How good the wine is will depend on your knowledgeability and how much you can afford. Don't try anything too unusual for this meal—absolutely no blueberry, plum or sparkling red wine. And don't spend fifteen dollars on a bottle unless you really know what you're getting; if he knows about wine, it will seem pretentious, and if he doesn't, it's a waste.

In white wines, stick to Chablis, Pouilly-Fuissé (or Fumé), Rhine wines and Moselles. Don't get rosé unless you're sure he likes it. Most people prefer either red or white. In red wines, you're always safe with all but the lowest-priced Beaujolais or Chateauneuf-du-Pape. For vintage wines, consult the chart that should be hanging in your liquor store. Don't go by label alone; the finest wine can taste like vinegar if it's too young. For example, a 1969 Burgundy is the best you can buy, but a Bordeaux of the same year is very risky.

Whatever you serve, don't make a fuss. Now is not the time to try out a fantastic recipe with twenty ingredients. And don't serve a great Russian feast or mounds of dumplings if you are looking for some after-dinner entertainment.

What you wear will depend on what you've got, in both senses: your wardrobe and your figure. Now is a perfect time to go without underwear, if you can afford to. If your breasts look pretty without a bra, leave it off. If you're comfortable without underpants, don't wear them. But if you'll be self-conscious, it's not worth it. Don't ever go without underwear just because you think that's a sexy thing to do, if it makes you feel uncomfortable. If you always need a bra, then wear a bra always, no matter what the situation. (Though you might want to get one of the soft, sheer bras that give you an unconstructed look.)

On such a night, I'd wear a cashmere caftan that molds (*not* sticks) to the body and is comfortable, soft and feminine. It's long-sleeved and buttons down to the waist, but there's space between the buttons, so it looks cut out down the front. I'm elegant at dinner, I can curl up in it, take it off, put it on, and it doesn't give away any secrets.

To me, subtlety is important at such a time. Both the atmosphere and the way you present yourself should be subtle. Subtlety is a way of letting him know you're available without actually saying it, without being too obvious.

For a seduction, I might wear what I call my "surprise sexy number." I'd go to my favorite beige or white silk blouse, which is long sleeved and man-tailored, but unbuttoned by one or two buttons more than it should be. It's not obvious. It's tucked in enough so that nothing shows—except at certain moments, when you may lean forward to let him light your cigarette, or to listen closely to something he has to say. You're giving out a message, but not screaming it. If you're nude under the silk, he'll know it. But you're giving him hints; you're using gentle persuasion instead of dragging him to your lair.

The most effective way of dressing is freely and as minimally as you can. If you understate your intentions, you'll be more provocative, and you'll also never have to deal with an out-and-out rejection.

Of course, as I said before, what you do and what you wear will depend on the man and on your expectations. If what you're looking for is a quick seduction of a passing plumber, then I don't see why you should bother putting anything on. Just call him up, and when he arrives at the door, open it *au naturel*. He'll certainly get the point and either be willing to go along or not. That's my guess, anyway— I'll have to admit I've never done it. Of course, you might be embarrassed if the person at the door turns out to be a Jehovah's Witness or a Bible salesman, but you *could* try convincing him you're practicing a new religion.

If the man who's coming to dinner is someone you want to see again, if he's the man of your dreams, of your life or even of the hour, then I

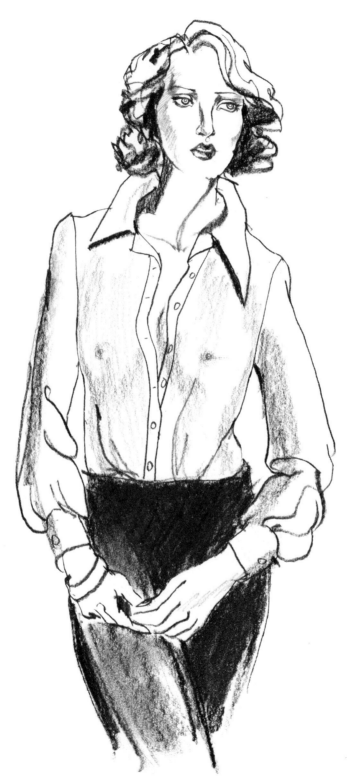

Here's my "surprise sexy number."

would recommend a little more discretion. If you're hoping for a pro-
longed relationship with him, you'll have time in the future to wear
outrageous little outfits or nothing at all. It's always better to be suggestive than too obvious. That's the charm of flirtation, after all. You
play with words, eyes and body, never pinning anything down exactly,
and at the same time lightly suggesting all of it. That game gives
pleasure to both of you. You flirt for your own satisfaction as much
as for his. When you dress for a seduction, let your appearance convey
the same subtle suggestiveness as a look of the eye or words with
double meanings.

If the situation is reversed, and *he's* the one planning the seduction,
you have to decide first of all whether or not you want to be seduced.
If not, you might decline the invitation. But if you're stuck with it and
there's no way out, and you've already invoked the death of close
relatives six times, then choose clothes and create a situation that obviously say no. Wear nonseductive clothes—high-necked, long-sleeved—
that don't reveal the body. Button up. And if you have nothing at all
that doesn't make you look desirable, the only possible recourse may
be to munch garlic before you meet him.

If he's planning it and you're delighted, dress as though it were your
idea too. It is, after all. The cashmere caftan and the man-tailored
shirt are just as good at his place as at yours. If you're going out
for dinner, wear anything that's soft and subtle, shows your body
when you move and is easy to get out of. Clothes that open down
the front are very suggestive, and so is anything in a very sheer (but
not transparent) fabric. Look like a lady in the restaurant, even if
you plan to turn into something else later.

The Morning After

Rosy-fingered dawn finds you curled up happily beside him. Marvelous.
You have to be in the office in an hour, and yesterday's clothes remain

where they landed when flung in ecstasy. Or they're hung neatly in the closet. In any case, they're yesterday's clothes, either what you put on for an evening out or what you were wearing at the office yesterday before you freshened up your makeup, dabbed your perfume and met him in the restaurant.

You could call in sick, but you have a nine-thirty appointment, and it's important. What to do?

The answer, for me at least, is never to get into such a situation. My standard rule is: if I'm going to be dressed in anything that's an after-six outfit, or if I'm meeting him directly from the office, I don't go to the guy's house—he comes to mine. Let *him* worry about leaving my apartment in a tuxedo at nine o'clock in the morning. I'm not going to worry about leaving his apartment in an evening gown at breakfast time.

I also would never want to be obvious enough to go back to the office next day in the same outfit I had on the day before. The only possibility is carrying an overnight bag. But it might seem a little too obvious if you meet him at a restaurant or arrive at his place carrying a suitcase.

It really isn't practical to take a complete change of clothes with you to work every day, just in case something good crops up. If you have a regular relationship with the man, you could leave a few outfits at his place, and he'll keep a few at yours. But if it's not that kind of relationship, or if it's a new and wonderful surprise, then have him come to you.

If it's *completely* surprising, and you find yourself in his bed at two in the morning, set the alarm for a time early enough to allow you to go home and change. And if he's in *your* bed, don't be offended if he does the same. You might even suggest it; he'll probably love you for your concern about him.

Dressing Up for Fun

When you know each other well, and particularly if you've been married or living together for years, it can be marvelous fun to wear something absolutely crazy. You don't have to be the Total Woman and greet your husband at the door wrapped in plastic, or wear a different costume every night, but once in a while something outrageous might be good for both of you.

You might buy one set of extraordinary underwear, like lacy and crotchless bikinis, black garters or a sheer bra with the nipples cut out—Frederick's-of-Hollywood kind of garments, dramatically and obviously meant for sex. Or a black lace jumpsuit that covers all of you except that one strategic area, or some other crazy little peekaboo whatnot.

It can be important to a relationship to come up with little surprises now and then. I don't advise it until and unless you know the guy well; otherwise you'll make him think you're something different than you really are. He might pigeonhole you into that costume, when for you it was just a frothy moment.

It's also important that you do this to make *both* of you happy. If you're doing it just for *him*, forget it. Do it for him only if you're doing it for yourself as well. Experiment with costumes—let yourself go. It was fun dressing up when you were little, and it might turn out to be even more fun now that you're a big girl. Try the high-black-boots routine, or the harem number. If you don't like it, you never have to do it again. On the other hand, you won't know till you've tried and you might end up surprising yourself, or both of you.

Getting out of yourself in these ways can enliven a marriage (or long relationship) and keep it young. The day a woman stops having a sense of play, puts aside all possibility of excitement or novelty and says, "I'm a mother first," or some such thing, is the day her marriage starts to dry up and crumble. Even the most exquisite cake is nothing when it's stale, and neither is a tart. Freshness is always important.

Greet your husband in Frederick's-type attire and see what happens. I'd make sure the children are away or tucked in bed asleep before doing this, otherwise you might be embarrassed by a small voice calling attention to the fact that your underwear has a hole in it or that you forgot to put your clothes on.

But let there be times for the two of you without the children. A marriage of five, ten, twenty years needs to be charged by a sexy, romantic atmosphere now and then.

If you're not married, dressing up can be a way of finding out how basically sensual the man is. It's also a way of letting him know about your sensuality, and it's a good means of finding out if you're suited (pardon the pun!) for each other.

As far as I'm concerned, anything at all is okay between a man and a woman as long as they're both happy doing it and aren't embarrassed or uncomfortable. I think it's a mistake to let a man convince you to become involved in anything that makes you uncomfortable. On the other hand, you won't know how you feel about it until you try.

If you want to costume yourself but are not sure how the man would take it, you can ask him. If your modesty prevents you, try going with him to a costume party (or give one yourself) and show him your fantasies in a less private way. (You'll also find out about his!)

There's no need to wear an out-and-out masquerade if you don't want to. But the one pair of lacy, open bikinis, the little patch of body painting or the silver stilettos can provide just that tiny pinch of something to spice up your life.

"Let's Get Away from It All"

Whether it's your first honeymoon or your twentieth, right after the wedding or ten years later, premarital or postmarital, this is a time when *everything* counts. It may be an overnight or weekend escape to a small hotel or a romantic splurge on the Isle of Capri; in either case, the two of you will be alone together most of the time, and your minds may be running along the same one track.

Whatever you wear should be pretty and comfortable, nonbinding, soft and easy to remove. If you meant to lose ten pounds for this occasion and you haven't, feel loose and live with it. Don't try to conceal the excess in girdles or support hose. Don't even take along any underwear that controls or constructs the body. Instead of support hose, take the sheerest, most delicate nylons you own. Or go out and buy a pair. As you pack, remember: Whatever goes on is sure to come off.

You'll be spending a lot of time in and around bed, so take sleepwear that isn't just for sleeping. Even if you're just going for the weekend, take a couple of nightgowns (or *very* sexy, feminine pajamas) and a lovely peignoir. Leave your "old reliables" at home; if your robe is comfortable and nothing else, get one that's comfortable and a lot more.

This is the greatest opportunity in the world for wearing the most luscious, luxurious, delectable night clothes you own or would like to own: lacy waltz gowns, short baby dolls in a very sheer fabric, ending at the top of the thigh over tiny panties; a marvelous old-fashioned satiny gown reaching to the floor, with lace trimming. If you have a little mad money saved, splurge on the most sensational, most elegant, sexiest, feminine nightdress you can find.

Choose it in your favorite color—whatever looks best on you. A black negligee may be the quintessence of sexiness, but black is only beautiful if you look good in black. The same gown may suit you even more deliciously in white—or ivory, or peach or pale blue. A combination gown-and-peignoir set can be devastating, particularly if one garment plays into the other. A long beige satin gown with tiny straps and delicate lace appliqué can't possibly be improved upon, except by a matching peignoir in beige lace with touches of satin, long sleeves tight at the wrist and a nipped-in waist.

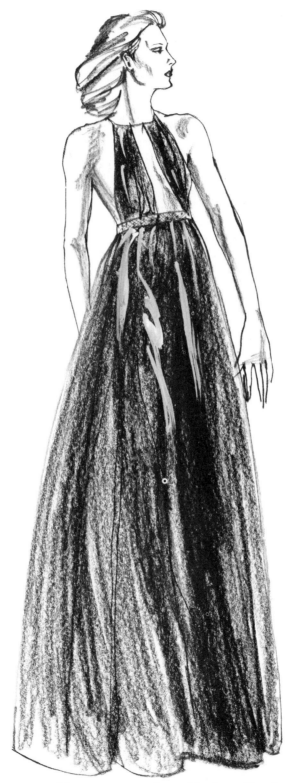

Is anything more sexy than a black negligee?

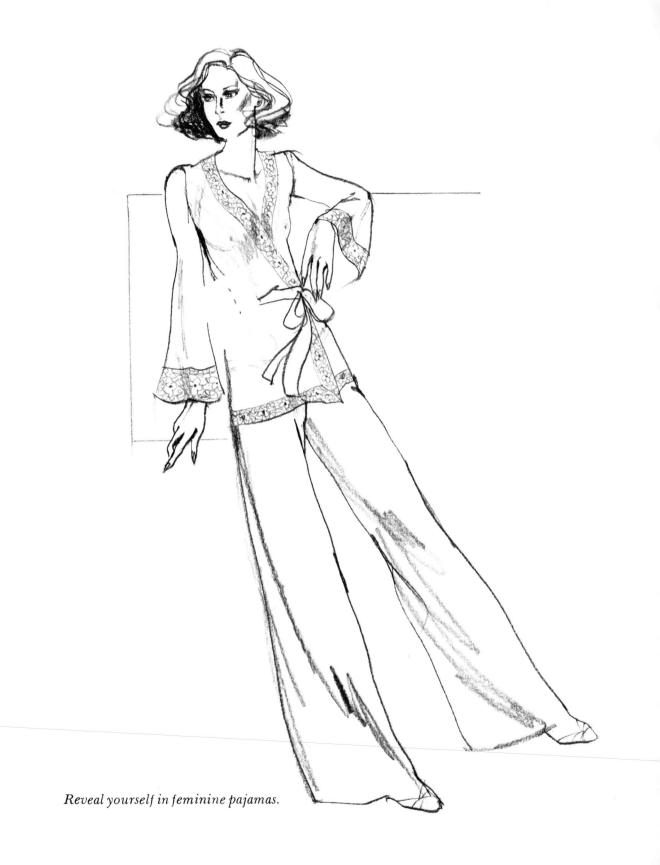

Reveal yourself in feminine pajamas.

You'll wear the robe for effect or room service, or both. Make sure it goes well with all the night clothes you're taking along, and wear slippers that match the whole ensemble.

You'll want your skin to be as touchable and irresistible as possible, so be sure to take along a super body lotion with minimal (preferably no) fragrance. Then you can spray your favorite scent strategically around your body and dab perfume wherever you want a longer-lasting effect. Your hair should be brushed out, clean and shining. Forget hair spray, even if you use it regularly. Imagine reaching out to ruffle his hair and finding your fingers caught in something hard and sticky!

With your makeup, use your best discretion. You know how you look without it, and you know if you want to take the chance to leave it off. If you think your man will be shocked and stunned to see you bare-faced, then wear the makeup or change the man. If you do wear a lot of makeup to bed, think how you'll look in the morning. Green eyeshadow is not lovely on the nose, and black mascara has never given a dewy look to someone's cheek.

You're probably best off with just a touch of mascara at the end of the lashes, to give depth to the eye. Apply very little, and use waterproof mascara. Touch your cheeks with blush-on to look healthy and glowing if *he* hasn't made you look that way already. Moisten your lips with a gloss or a pale, dewy lipstick that won't be noticeable when it comes off. A fresh, dewy mouth is very sexy; a dry one isn't.

Don't be uptight about makeup. If you add a touch to lashes and lips when you brush your teeth, that should be enough. If you feel you can't risk letting him see you without makeup, if you think you have to set the alarm for 4:00 A.M. so you can do a quick touch-up under the covers, something's probably wrong in your relationship. For the first two years of my first marriage, I did that kind of thing. It's not a very relaxed way to start a relationship. If you can bear the man, bare your face.

You'll want to bare your body too, but perhaps not at first. A nude body is often very beautiful, but leading up slowly to that moment when you uncover it all is wonderfully exciting. A body that's strategically covered is usually more provocative than nudity.

This is perhaps one reason why many men become attracted to older women. An older woman is less likely to have a perfect young body, but much more apt than a young woman to use those little enticements that make a woman seem beautiful and devastating. The older woman will wear a simple, gorgeous nightgown that makes the most of her skin tone or her eyes. She'll wear delicate little bed slippers and a regal marabou bed jacket. She'll create an atmosphere of sexiness and loveliness that will really excite a man. At the time of making love, no man is concerned with the perfect young body.

Few women, even when they're very young, have absolutely perfect bodies anyway. It's most wonderful to show your body at the point when it's most desired. Really: The partly concealed body will arouse more interest than stark nudity. Think of Salome and her veils. If she'd left them off, she might never have gotten ahead.

"Please Come to Our Little Den of Iniquity"

If you're invited for a group swing, don't immediately reach for your petticoats and your square-dancing skirt. Nowadays such events rarely have a caller, and your petticoats would be sure to get in the way (not to mention the laced bodice!).

For better or worse, orgies are not part of my experience, and I include in that category all kinds of "swinging" evenings requiring more than two participants. However, since this book should serve as a dressing guide to the modern woman in all likely (and unlikely) circumstances, I'd like to pass on a few pointers I've learned from friends or acquaintances more adventurous than I.

Number 1. Don't wear anything that binds or leaves marks on the body. It's very unattractive.

Number 2. Omit stockings and underwear, if possible. Not only do they leave marks on the body when they come off—they're also likely to get in your way and be unnecessarily cumbersome.

Number 3. Wear sexy clothes. They should be very body-conscious (like the guests) and should emphasize your best features. Whatever clings is fine. This is a perfect occasion to wear any see-through garments you own, though even in this situation the see-through blouse should not merely be a soft windowpane, but should rather be suggestive. If everything's laid out for inspection, some people will stop with window-shopping and never come in.

Number 4. Sew name tapes on all articles of personal property; it's easier to reclaim them afterward.

After the End

If you're happy about your divorce, wear a fire-engine red suit. If you're sad, you really won't think about what to wear for the occasion.

I know there are women who go to Reno or Mexico or wherever for their divorce and treat it like a vacation, or a husband-hunting safari. They'll pack their most devastating outfits to get a man, or to get even. But I, for one, don't think that the occasion of your divorce is a highly sexual or fashion-conscious time.

Generally speaking, I think most women find divorce an extremely difficult time. The sooner you can overcome the traumatic experience you've gone through, the better. Change is very important now. Since your life has already been changed in a very significant way, it's best to remove as many signs of the old life as possible.

By that I mean moving to another apartment, another town, another part of the country. Changing jobs, if possible—to start again as a new person. It's a time to go back to school, to take up an interest or a talent you've ignored for too long—and to get new clothes. This is really the one time in life when I'd go out and get a totally new wardrobe. New everything, or as many new garments as I could afford.

Otherwise, you keep being thrown back to memories which might be very painful. The blue dress was his favorite. You take it off and put on the yellow suit. That's what you wore boarding the plane when the two of you went to Europe, and the stewardess spilled some wine on it, and he mopped it up and said he liked the pattern it made and . . .

Or you look at the long brown skirt you wore New Year's Eve; was it really only this past New Year's, such a short time ago. . . ?

Or those bikini underpants he loved, calling himself the fastest hand on the drawer . . .

Almost every item you own will carry memories, and unless you're extremely strong, or *really* happy about the divorce, or if you can't afford to get new clothes, I'd definitely advise selling, trading, giving away or just throwing out your married wardrobe.

Buy the clothes that will bring you out the most. You can now get all the things you wanted but couldn't wear when you were with him because he didn't like the style or color. Get bright clothes, even if your tendency now is to wear black or somber colors. For your own emotional well-being, it's important to wear outfits that give off some gaiety, with brightness, to put you in the most sunshiny mood possible.

Above all, don't dress like a nun or a penitent. Your clothes can help you feel better about yourself, and the better you feel, the more you'll be interested, not just in what you wear, but in everything about you. Don't be mourning the past with your actions or your appearance. One aspect of your life may be over, but another is certainly beginning, so pick yourself up, freshen your face and start all over again.

Get a new hair style, have yourself made up, buy something in a color you've never worn before. If you have children, it's even more important for you to look cheerful and attractive. They'll probably feel confused and unhappy about the divorce and will take their cues from you as to how to behave now. Your appearance will reassure them and tell them to keep their sunny side up.

Even if you and he were never married, the ending can be extremely painful. Perhaps even more than the ex-wife, you'll have to learn to stop regretting. Start with your appearance, make it as attractive as you can. You're then making a statement of strength: This is who I am, and I will continue to be my own person. Others will respect you for it, and may even love you.

Dressing for Men

I used to dress *for* men—or *for* women—but I don't anymore. Now, I basically dress to present the part of my personality that I want people to see. But while I'm expressing that aspect of my personality, I'm also displaying my individual style. When my clothes are free, flowing and sensual because I'm feeling that way, they'll still be understated. That's my personality, and any mood I happen to be in will still be influenced by it.

Some women, I've noticed, change their style of dressing with a new boyfriend or husband. The woman who does this is obviously playing a game. She's trying to present a personality different from her real self because she thinks this is what the man wants. This is a bad policy, and one that will almost certainly get her in trouble. Once she's made the conquest, starts to relax and become herself again, she's suddenly making a totally different kind of statement.

It's very important that women remember how much they're saying about themselves through their clothes, and then consciously make the decision about whether or not to play games in the early stages.

The same is true within an established relationship. You've got to decide how far you'll let yourself be influenced by him—or you can be led to making *his* statement about you instead of your own.

If I put on something I adore and the man I'm dating or am married to doesn't like it, I won't wear it again when I'm with him, but I will definitely continue to wear it with other people or on my own. That's true of me now. Ten years ago if I had put on an outfit for the first time and if my husband had said, "I don't like that on you," I would never have been able to wear it again. His reaction would have destroyed it for me, and I wouldn't have felt comfortable in it even when I was lunching with a girlfriend or whatever else I was doing.

I now feel strongly enough about who I am and what I want to project about myself that I'm no longer totally dependent on what the man in my life says. I'm less hung up with clothes in that sense, and I think most women today have come along the same route, and are more into who they are. They know that clothes, however important, don't necessarily *make* the man (or woman). Clothes bring out the personality and are an important aspect of it, but the old dependency on male approval no longer controls most women's decisions about their clothes.

The woman of today basically no longer cares if the bed isn't made first thing in the morning, or if the dishes aren't done immediately after breakfast. She doesn't want to be judged as a woman by outmoded yardsticks. The same goes for her clothes. She may play with old-fashioned "cutesy" and "sultry" outfits, but it's not where her head is really at. She dresses for the occasion, and to make her own statement, and though she may soften her outfit a little when she's with a man, she will not dress directly *for* him.

I dress for the occasion, but I never change my basic style. Even between the public and the private self there's no real split. We all have many facets. The public and the private you should both be part of who you are.

I see myself as giving the impression of a rather dignified, ladylike, business woman. That doesn't mean I'm not silly or sensuous or provocative or many other things that have nothing to do with the picture I present to a lot of people. I can shift to an almost see-through blouse or a backless, practically frontless dress, as long as it's tasteful and not too obvious; I can get away with it as part of my general style.

It's right and healthy that our choice of what to wear will depend on where we're going and what we intend to do, rather than on the man. He too, after all, is guided by the occasion.

The limits to independence are dictated by common sense. When a man who's very important to you dresses in a way you can't stand, it's a good idea to tell him. He would probably tell you if he dislikes something you have on, and if you care about him, it's best to be honest. Otherwise, chances are you'll become more and more aggravated by the way he presents himself until you won't feel good being with him. You might even end by breaking up with him because he'll be constantly antagonizing you, though without knowing it. He picks you up for a dinner date and is wearing that same absolutely hideous purple tie with a herringbone jacket that you hated when you first saw it six wearings ago. Your heart sinks, and you already dread your entrance into the restaurant.

You're better off saying from the beginning, "I adore you, but that tie's got to go." Or something like it. What you say will depend on the relationship you have with him and on the kind of person he is. Can he handle it? Will he see your criticism as an attack on himself? Or can you frame your criticism in a constructive statement?

You can tell him how you feel about his clothes without making a personal attack if you're humorous about it and present it almost as a joke. You might say, "I saw my grandmother getting hit by a truck of that same color . . ." Or: "I know it's very fashionable, but pea soup always disagreed with me . . ."

However you say it, make sure he gets the message. You don't want to cower every time you walk into a public place with him. But be fair. If you expect him to change his clothes, or not to wear his beloved polka-dot dinner jacket when he's with you, then you must be prepared to accept his criticism or suggestions.

I think we've all learned to become more honest and more ourselves. We don't have to dress *for* a man, or he *for* us. But we don't have to dress *against* each other either.

5

The Sporting Life

At the Game

When the mustard's dripping, the beer foaming and there's a tied score at the top of the ninth, you're not going to worry about your clothes. You shouldn't have to; you're at the game for fun, excitement, letting go, being a kid again, or screaming till you're hoarse.

Particularly if you're going with the kids, chances are something will be upset beside the score. And you'd spoil the fun if you made a fuss over the stain. If you know you'll be part of an excited, milling crowd, your first rule should be to wear something very washable. If you own anything stainless, wear it. A jacket made of PVC can be cleaned on the spot with a napkin dipped in water.

For the grandstand, for Coney Island, or for your child's Little League game, it's a good idea to wear jeans, unless they don't suit you or you find them too hot. Short of tuning your car engine or unstopping the toilet, this is the most informal situation that you can possibly be in. Be comfortable and wear clothes you never have to think about, whether you're sitting on the grass (for the Little League game) or on benches that people have just walked over. Tie a kerchief around your

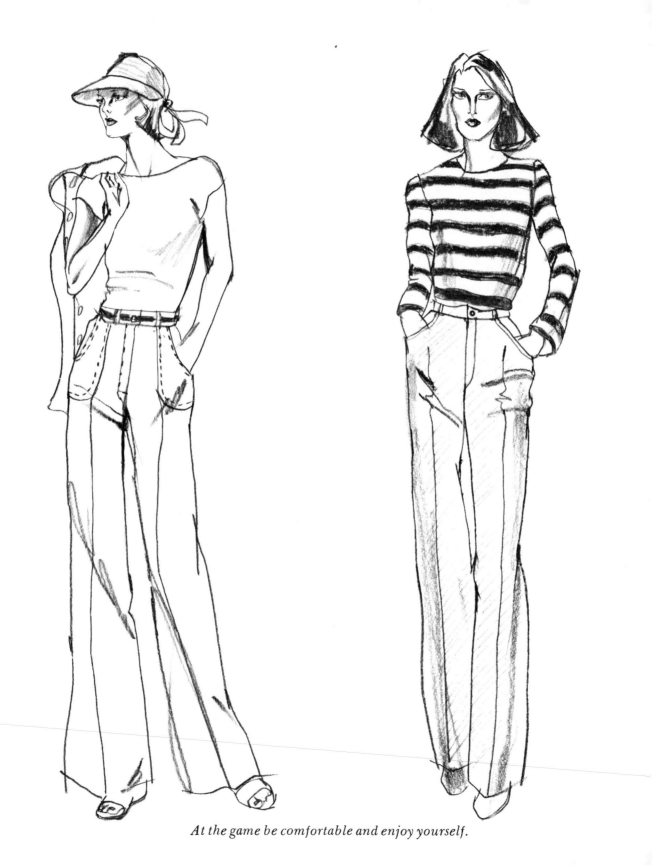

At the game be comfortable and enjoy yourself.

hair or wear a play hat if you'll be sitting in the sun a long time. A floppy straw hat, a fedora, a cap with visor are all good to keep out the sun and also don't look as though you're trying to make a fashion statement.

If it's a night game, you'll remember to take an extra sweater, jacket or stole. No matter how hot it is when you start out, by eleven o'clock at night you can be frozen to the spot, right? For cold-weather sports, like football, wear the warmest coat you own, wrap a long woolen scarf around your neck and tuck it into the coat; cover your head and ears with a woolen cap. The old-fashioned raccoon coat is marvelous—so is any fun fur you have. If your warmest coat is a sable, wear your next-warmest. If you're sitting on the bench looking as though you were expecting fashion photographers any minute, you'll be an object of embarrassment or ridicule. Nobody will believe you care about the sport at all.

Your most informal dressing (in summer, denim skirt and top, culottes, sundress) is appropriate to all games where you know you'll be in a grandstand, bleachers or on the ground. The few exceptions to this rule are generally European sports—bullfighting, for instance, where jeans would not be appropriate no matter how far away from the bullring you're sitting—and those sports that are considered more formal like polo.

How formally you dress for a sports event will depend on two things: where you sit and how important or glamorous the event is. If you drop by Belmont on an ordinary weekday, don't change unless you're coming from an elegant luncheon, in which case you've already missed the first two races, and it might be better just to stop off at OTB this day. But if you go to watch the Belmont Stakes in an owner's box, put on a dress or suit. You can dress as for a tea party and put on a Southern belle kind of hat if you want to. You can even get away with little white gloves and a Scarlett O'Hara type dress. Don't wear such an outfit, however—even for the Stakes—if you're going in on General Admission.

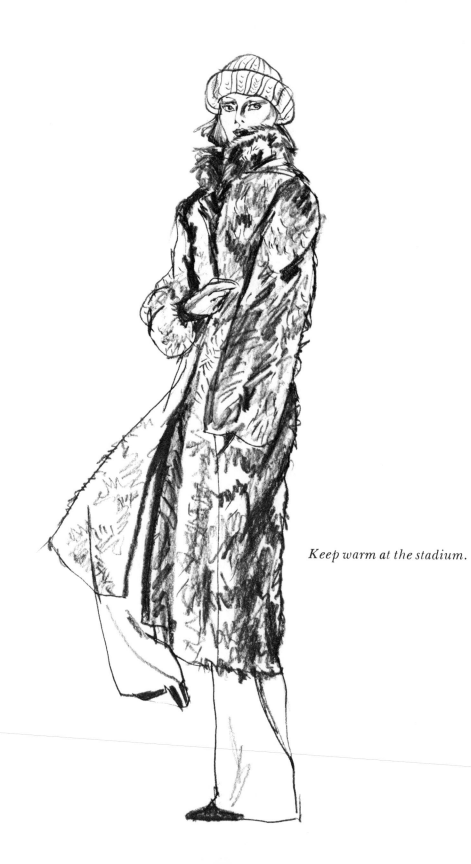

Keep warm at the stadium.

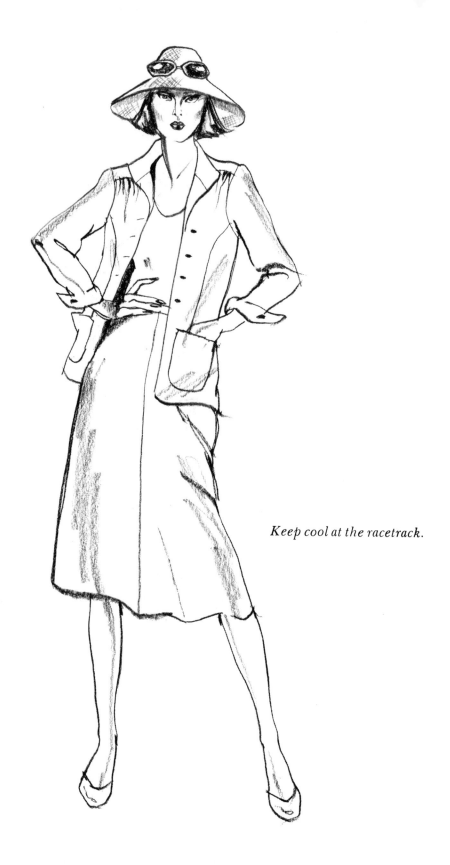

Keep cool at the racetrack.

For tennis at Forest Hills, or an exhibition match played for charity or a political candidate, wear anything from a knit suit to a pants suit.

If formal dressing is required for any sports event, you'll know in advance. This would happen if you are specially invited and the invitation specifies black tie. Or it may be formal if the event is combined with another—if you've been invited to dine at the race track, for instance, and it will be a formal celebration. Then you dress for the dinner, not the horses.

Generally, though, if the event is out of doors and during the daytime, you wear daytime, outdoorsy, informal clothes. European sports events tend to be dressier than ours, and if you're going to the Ascot or to Lord's for the cricket matches, ask your host or escort for advice. You don't want to be overdressed if he has inexpensive seats. On the other hand, it would be downright rude for you, a foreigner, to appear in pants when the ladies around you are behatted and begloved, and in their best silks.

When you're traveling somewhere because of an event, take along party clothes. If you're going to Kentucky, say, for the Derby, pack clothes to wear at parties the evening before, and perhaps for the victory party afterward. Pack soft, clinging garments that hang out when you hang them up. Tunics—short or long—are excellent. Take things in light or bright colors, in thin fabrics. A scarlet crepe tunic with a long skirt of the same color, or with loose, soft pants to match, would be a sensational outfit. Or choose romantic, long, flowing clothes. Consider taking a pastel Mexican wedding dress, a column of electric blue, off the shoulder with a matching stole; and a short cocktail dress, well-fitting and unfussy but in a wonderful material like silk. Chiffon, organza or batiste are marvelous fabrics for the clothes you take to Louisville. Be dreamy and romantic in the evening, but for the race itself, wear something crisp and chic. A dress with jacket is excellent, in white with navy trimming (or navy with white) and a touch of bright red or kelly green in a scarf or belt.

The Sporting Life

Whether it's Louisville or some place else where a sports event is the occasion for parties and festivity, let the frills and folds and long skirts come out at night, but wear bright, clean sports clothes for the actual event. This rule is good for the opening of the Olympic games too, or any other great moment in the world of sports.

If you want better seats than you think he's planning to get, you might practice the art of gentle persuasion. Instead of wearing jeans or a denim skirt to a game—which right away announce that you'd be willing to sit on the ground—wear your crisp navy and white suit. It's still casual, and appropriate for most games, but it does carry a message of longing for better seats. He may not be conscious of why he's changing his mind at the last moment and asking for loge instead of grandstand, but he's getting the signal. Your clothes are saying you want to be somewhere clean, and he'll probably want to show off the good-looking chic woman beside him. This is a quieter and more effective way of manipulating the situation than coming right out and asking him to get better seats. If you're in jeans and sweat shirt, watch out! He might try to change his box seats for the bleachers.

Sports clothes, the pride of American designing, are intended for spectator sports. They're hardly ever the clothes you'd actually play in, but they're perfect for watching the Big Game. Always make sure you carry a stole or some cover-up in case the weather turns or the wind comes whistling down. And if there's any chance you'll be spending the afternoon out in the sun, wear a hat to protect your face. A kerchief is fine for protecting the hair, and essential if your hair is artificially colored, but it won't protect your face, and hours of baking in the sun will not make you look cool and attractive. It's also not healthy; too much exposure isn't good for any kind of skin.

Remember also: If you're in the bright sun, makeup should be very subtle. You want a natural outdoors look, and hard black lines in bright sunlight will make you look harsh, older and out of place. Try using

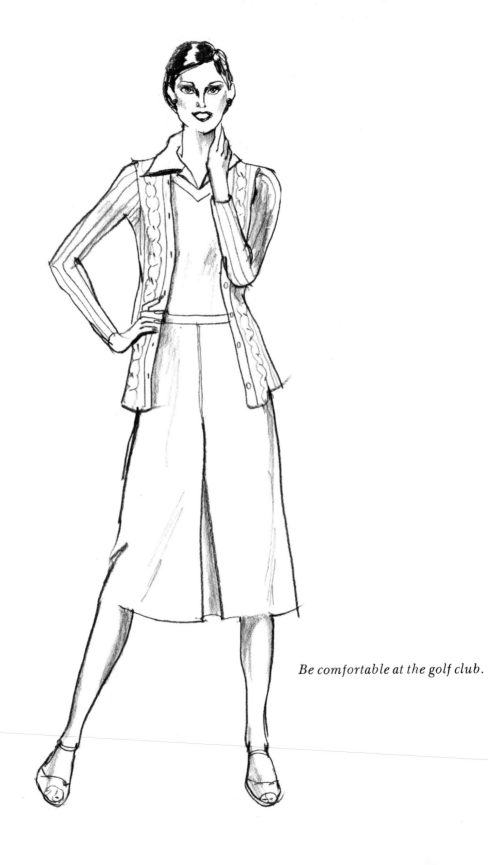

Be comfortable at the golf club.

one of those mirrors with controlled lighting that permit you to apply makeup according to the kind of light you'll be in. Or check your makeup out of doors before you leave, to make sure the mellow brown in the bathroom mirror doesn't look like coal in the sunlight.

Whatever the game is, be comfortable and sporty. There's no reason why you can't look pretty and feminine as well, but let the added touches show up in accessories—a straw hat, straw bag, a scarf around the neck or at the waist, chalk-white jewelry or a colorful rope belt. Otherwise, show you're a sport by wearing casual, no-nonsense, no-fuss sportswear. And don't forget your sunglasses.

Play Ball

Most games and sports require professional equipment and standard uniforms, though if you're not professional, you have a lot of leeway in what you wear. Generally, for whatever sport it is, make sure your hair is neat and out of your way. If it's long, tie it up in a ponytail or braids or a very simple upsweep. Use a headband, ribbon or kerchief— unless there's special headwear appropriate to the sport.

Use makeup very sparingly; a touch of lipstick, blush-on and mascara is all you'll probably need. Use a moisturizer on your skin instead of foundation, which will probably show in the sunlight. Keep clean and cool; use scent and talc. Grooming and neatness are essential for any sport. Whatever you're playing has its rules, and if you look sloppy on the court or green, you'll give an amateurish impression. Your own game will probably suffer too. Your appearance is a statement to the outside world, but it is equally a statement you make to yourself. If your hair's in your face, or your socks are bagging around the ankles, you'll be less inclined to play your best game than if everything is under control. Even if you're a beginner, try to look as though you knew the game. It will help you learn it faster.

Make sure your playing clothes are clean and pressed. If you're going in for a sport with any regularity at all, have at least two outfits so you can always change into a fresh one. After a game, your clothes will be sticky and slightly crumpled; you probably won't want to wear them a second time without a washing in between. For that reason, they should be machine-washable and durable. Think of your tennis or golf outfits as though they were garments you were buying for toddlers—they'll be in the washing machine more than any other clothes you own.

Invest in footwear. Whatever sport it is, and whatever type shoes are required, get comfortable ones that won't slip. It's not enough to get well-fitting shoes; you have to find shoes with *perfect* fit. Otherwise your game will suffer.

If you're playing a game out of doors, remember to take along a sweater—or a sweat shirt or stole—for afterward; again, make it something highly washable. Even if the day is warm, you'll be cooling off after the game and will almost invariably need to put on an additional something.

Sit, run, jump, swing in the dressing room. Test your sports clothes before you buy them through actions that will show you how the garment feels and looks during play. Anything binding or constricting is useless.

Following are general guidelines, including some specific suggestions, for most of the games you might play.

Tennis. White tennis shoes are imperative, no matter what else you wear. Without them, you won't be allowed on the court. Buy white ones, even though sneakers are sneakers in any color. If you wear red tennis shoes, you'll be calling attention to your feet and people will watch you closely for mistakes. If you wear gag footwear, people will be expecting you to fall flat on your face.

Wear white tennis socks—either cotton bobby socks or the little terry numbers with a pom-pom at the back of the heel to keep them

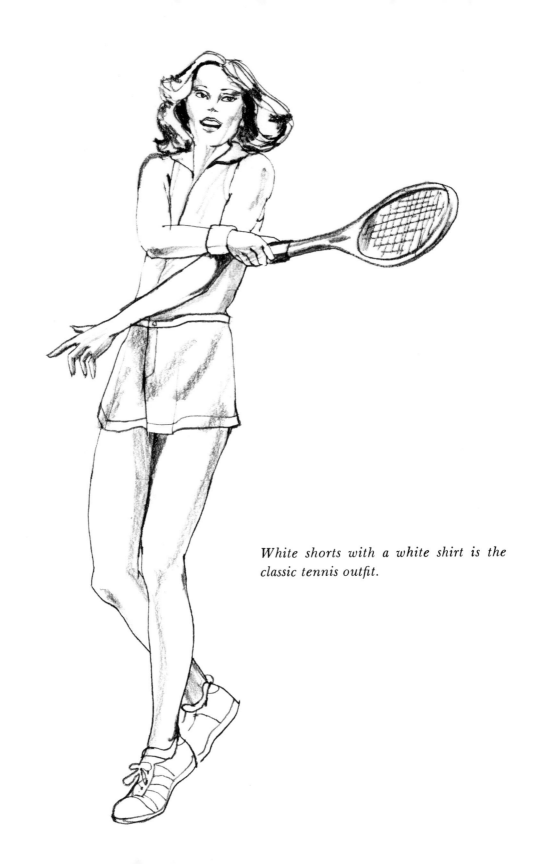

White shorts with a white shirt is the classic tennis outfit.

from sliding. Nylon or any other slippery fabric is not good. The socks should stay in place, prevent chafing and soak up perspiration.

If you're a beginner, get the traditional white tennis shorts instead of a tennis dress. If you give up the game later, you can wear the shorts with colored tops. Buy a white cotton shirt or T-shirt; again, it can always be worn for other occasions. If you don't want to be all in white, a navy top is the next best choice. Don't wear a patterned top, unless you prefer an exhibition to the sport. White shorts and matching T-shirt are the tennis player's classic outfit, and it's always good to have at least one set.

Outfits specifically made for tennis—little dresses, skirts or short jumpsuits—are extremely attractive. But if you're buying a tennis dress, don't let your first consideration be sexiness. The short, loose dress with panties peeking out from underneath (if the dress doesn't come with panties, go to a dance store and get the leotard kind you wear over tights) are provocative in themselves. When you're moving around on the court, the sexy nipped-in number in a size smaller than you should wear is likely to be more embarrassing than enticing. The dress can be in any color but have at least one in white, just in case. Some courts in this country and abroad will not let you play if you're in anything but white.

A headband that matches your outfit gives you a cool, professional look. Or wear a cotton—*not* silk—scarf that's fresh and starched. A tennis outfit is probably the most feminine of all sports uniforms; don't exaggerate its cuteness or you'll be invited to donate your court time to serious players.

The great tennis stars develop their own style of dressing. But they perform in front of the public eye and television cameras; their uniform doubles as an entertainer's outfit. It is also their everyday business clothing, and they may choose occasional variety. On the whole, though, even Billie Jean King and Chris Evert dress for the sport and not the spectators. And we look at their game instead of their clothes.

Golf. Again, start with shoes, and wear the same kind of socks you'd wear for tennis. Decide if you'll be more comfortable in shorts or a skirt. Either way, your hemline will be at about the same place—well above your knees, for freedom of movement, and well below your groin, for tastefulness. As with tennis, sexiness will show in the way you move your body. Crotch-hugging shorts and micro-minis are out of place on the green. Shorts should be Jamaica or Bermuda length.

Protect your skin against the sun with moisturizers and lotion. Wear a cotton hat with a little brim or visor if the sun is strong. Make sure your sunglasses don't fall off your nose and that your golf glove fits perfectly.

Wear a top that's loose and cool and won't constrict your swing in any way. Let all the swing be in your stroke: Keep your hair back and jewelry off, with the possible exception of a wristwatch.

Bowling. The only special clothes you need are bowling shoes, and you usually rent these at the alley. Make sure you're wearing cotton or athletic socks and that the shoes you rent are really your size.

Depending on whether it's day or evening—an after-school treat for the kids or a bowling party with dinner and drinks—you can wear anything from jeans to dress, but don't choose a dress more elaborate than any you'd wear to the office. Suits and costumes are not good for bowling and neither, obviously, is anything cut too tightly in the arm or across the chest. You don't want to have to stop in midroll because something just ripped.

For bowling you can, if you want, be more dressy than for most other sports. Jewelry is fine if it doesn't swing or clank. You can makeup for indoors, but don't overdo it; anything too fussy or obviously sexy looks as though you came along just for fun, not for the game.

Team sports. If you're a woman who plays baseball or basketball, you're individualistic enough to know exactly what to wear. If you're on a team, you'll be given a uniform or told exactly what to wear. If it's sandlot softball or volleyball in the gym or handball at the playground, just think about the game—the clothes will take care of themselves. If the belt's too tight, you'll loosen it or take it off. You'll put your jewelry in your handbag and roll up your flare jeans. If you've been asked to join a soccer game and you answer, "I'd love to, but what'll I wear?", you're probably better off just watching.

The country club day. Though it's tennis in the morning, followed by a dip in the pool, lunch on the terrace, a game of golf, another dip, cocktails, dinner and dancing, you don't have to take along a steamer trunk. Pack everything you need in a small bag. Chances are you'll be keeping some of your equipment at the club in any case.

Think in terms of clothes that don't wrinkle. Choose knits and jerseys that you could even roll up into a ball, if you were so minded, and they'd still hang out while you took your shower.

A sundress or any simple summer outfit consisting of a skirt and top is fine for lunch. Take along a sweater, too. The restaurant will be air-conditioned, and you'll be particularly susceptible to the cold after a morning spent exerting yourself in the sun. For dinner or dancing, you can wear a long version of the sundress you had on at lunch—or a long skirt or loose, flowing pajama-type pants with a little top. Any of these will iron out by themselves in a few minutes and only need a few inches of packing space. Your sandals won't take much room either (flesh-colored ones will go with anything at all you might wear, day or evening), and jewelry goes into a side pocket or in your handbag. Your makeup and atomizer will be in your handbag already, and whatever sports clothes you need for the day should fit nicely into a satchel or overnight or flight bag.

Don't complicate your life by taking anything that will crease or need special care. A summer day at the club, on the beach or in a meadow should be light, simple and buoyant. Your look of health will brighten whatever you're wearing, and you should aim for the summer prettiness of wildflowers, not the cultivated look of hothouse roses.

Noncompetitive and Individual Sports

It's a good idea to have a leotard for exercising at home in case the doorbell rings and it's a Western Union messenger who's just stepped out of the past to bring you a telegram. Exercising or sunbathing in the nude is only advisable if you're willing to draw the blinds, ignore the door and forget about helicopters.

For most sports you do alone or with a companion, some form of dress is required or preferred, even in a heat wave.

Dawn people, up and raring to go at a time when most of us are hanging on to dreams for dear life and some of us are returning home in evening clothes, should have a warm, comfortable garment at hand to slip into for those hours before they'll have to dress for business or whatever else they will be doing. Even if your idea of jogging is once around the breakfast table, a jogging suit is a marvelous outfit to own. It's as comfortable as pajamas, though it doesn't look as though you've just gotten out of bed, and it's very attractive. It's the perfect thing to wear for most sports when the weather is cool, and it's ideal for crisp mornings when you walk the dog, get the paper, take your constitutional or, even, jog.

A jogging suit is basically sweat shirt and sweat pants, but you can now get them in a wide variety of styles, colors and fabrics. A light color is especially practical for year-round wear, including beach picnics on summer nights or as cozy cover-ups after a midnight or prebreakfast swim. They have an ensemble look, but are designed mainly for comfort and coziness. Don't buy one that's too tight, but don't let it be too loose either—or you may find, after a few washings, that they're slipping down faster than you can make it home.

You can wear a jogging suit for hiking, walking or bike riding. However, if the weather's too warm, or if you'll be stopping off some place for a bite to eat, you're probably better off in clothes that are just a

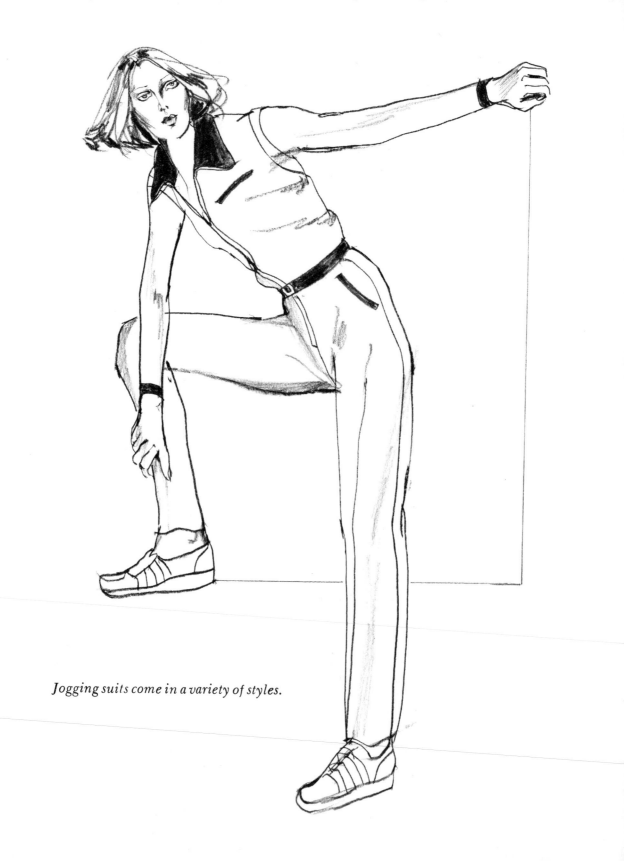

Jogging suits come in a variety of styles.

tiny bit more "dressy." They'll be loose, casual and comfortable, of course, and you'll wear good rubber-soled walking shoes or sneakers. For example, you can wear a wrap-around skirt and top or well-fitting jeans or culottes. When bike riding, remember not to wear long pants unless they're tight around the ankles. If they're wide, tuck the bottom of the pants leg into your sock, or tie a tiny wire around the ankle to hold the pants leg in place so that it won't get caught on the bike chain or in the gears.

Skirts of any kind are not suitable for bike riding. Culottes, though, are okay. If it's summer, and you decide to wear shorts, remember that your thighs will be exposed to the sun mercilessly, and I probably needn't mention that they are a delicate part of the body.

In New York I go bike riding in Central Park on weekends, when the park is closed to cars and the roads are reserved for cyclists. I wear blue jeans and sneakers with a sweater set or blouse and sweater. I'll wear a windbreaker if it's cold or windy. And this is one of the very few times in my life when I wear gloves. I always wear them biking, to protect my hands against calluses.

When you're out walking or hiking, protect yourself against insects, thorns, bushes and poison ivy by wearing long pants. If you wear shorts or a skirt, put on pretty knee-high stockings. Your knees may still get bitten or burned, but at least your ankles and calves will be smooth and protected.

It's a good idea to wear as many layers as you think you might need, instead of the one gorgeous ski sweater which is perfect in early morning coolness but unbearable at noon—or, conversely, the little tank top that's just right when you start out after lunch, but becomes a little cut-out among the goose pimples by the time you get home. A tank top with a cotton shirt over it, tucked into your pants or skirt, and a cardigan over that, provide you with alternatives for most weather changes. You can tie whatever you're not wearing around your shoulders, waist or hips, adding or peeling as the sun comes and goes, leaving the shirt

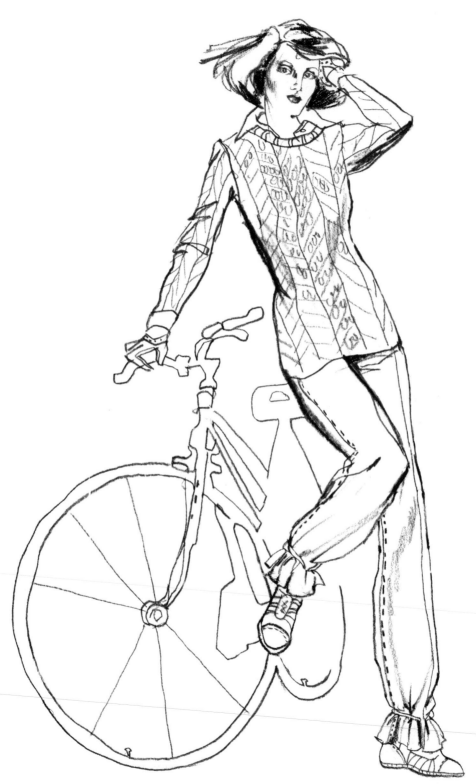

Protect your hands while bike riding and wear comfortable clothes.

unbuttoned with sleeves rolled up, or buttoned everywhere with open cardigan. This way you can comfortably take care of 30- to 40-degree temperature changes.

That's the best way to dress if you're a bird watcher, too. You may be up before the sun, and it's cold at owl-time. For bird watching, the best jacket to have is a lightweight army or safari type, with large pockets at the hip, smaller ones at the breast. It's the ideal jacket for a shutterbug too. If you need your hands for whatever equipment you're using, you won't want to carry a bag. Some bird watchers are photographers too and carry binoculars, cameras, special lenses and extra film, among other things. There's also the telescope for looking at water birds.

You'll want to carry your field guide in one pocket and your cigarettes, sunglasses, handkerchief in the other. Keys, money, driver's license and any other valuable items can go into one of the breast pockets and be buttoned in for safety. For bird watching, wear rubber-soled shoes and, if possible, earth colors or whatever affords you the best camouflage. In this activity, you want to be as unobtrusive as possible.

All the up-and-out people who like to greet the day, should provide for flexibility—clothes that will protect them against excessive sun, against cold or chills, and against rain. Nature is always changeable, and you must be ready to adapt to all her whims.

If you're cantering into day, posting in the dawn, you're a serious rider who owns serious riding gear and perhaps even the horse. Riding costumes are beautiful, on men as well as women. For the traditional English saddle, you'll need jodhpurs, a tailored shirt or turtleneck sweater, your riding jacket and boots. The riding cap is optional. If you look good in caps, wear it—it gives a marvelous total look. But if it doesn't suit you or is uncomfortable, leave it off.

If you ride regularly, go to a riding shop and buy the standard outfit. But if you've been invited for just one ride in the dawn, with champagne and strawberries afterward, you don't have to invest in the entire gear. Improvise by tucking your pants into walking boots, wear a tailored shirt or turtleneck sweater and put a blazer (or any sports jacket you own) over it.

For all specific sports outfits, go to a sports store. There you'll be equipped from head to toe, including the little details like socks, which you might ordinarily forget. Some sports outfits are so attractive you might want to wear them without ever actually going near the sport they were designed for. If you can afford it, go ahead. You can wear the tennis dress when you're marketing in the summer and the riding outfit, complete with crop, on a winter's evening for indoor sports with your man.

In the Swim

Forget about fashion. Choose the bathing suit that looks most stunning on you, and then get that style in a few colors. Leave bikinis, cut-outs, bottomless and topless suits to those who can afford to wear them without embarrassing everyone on the beach. You pick the suit that's meant for your figure.

Any woman with loose flesh around the middle, with sagging stomach or buttocks, should keep away from the two-piece or bikini as from the plague. The one-piece suit that's almost a tank suit will work to hold some of the loose flesh in and will produce a smooth line. In fact, almost everyone looks best in that kind of suit. No greater bathing suit has ever been designed than the one-piece tank-topped maillot. It's the classic black bathing suit—which can also be white, chocolate brown, almost any color. It can be loosely constructed for women who need support at the breasts, or totally unconstructed.

Years ago, suits were sometimes built like corsets, with heavy wiring and boning. This is an unhealthy and unattractive look, and I'm glad you can't find it anymore. The same goes for the "cute" little suits, with baby doll dresses or skirts. We've gotten further away from super-silly dressing on the beach. Beachwear is now basically streamlined and simple, and looks as though you can actually swim in it.

You'll want to elaborate on basic simplicity only if you have a figure defect that can comfortably be concealed by the addition. For instance, the woman with a very serious lower-hip or top-of-the-thigh problem could choose a tiny skirt to conceal a lot of ills. But she must still be very careful not to accomplish the opposite: calling attention to the defect by something that's obviously a cover-up.

Unless you won't be swimming in anything larger than a bathtub, make sure the suit will stay on you and be comfortable in the water. A fancy cut-out suit that doesn't stay up by itself will leave hideous strap marks at your neck or on your shoulders that destroy the look of other clothes you wear. Choose a suit with tiny little straps that can be hidden inside when you're tanning, then buttoned on or tied when you swim. Your suit has to serve two purposes, and there's no way in the world you can swim in the perfect tanning outfit. You need the straps to be comfortable in the water and legal coming out. But you don't want to walk around with tribal markings, either. So choose something that gives you the most out of both swimming and tanning.

If you're the kind of woman who doesn't care how she looks and you just want to get as much sun and water on your body as possible, you'll wear the absolute minimum. This depends on your ego, how concerned you are with your body. If I had a lot of excess weight, I wouldn't be caught dead in a bikini. No matter how much I wanted a suntan—I'd tell myself I should have thought of that before I got fat.

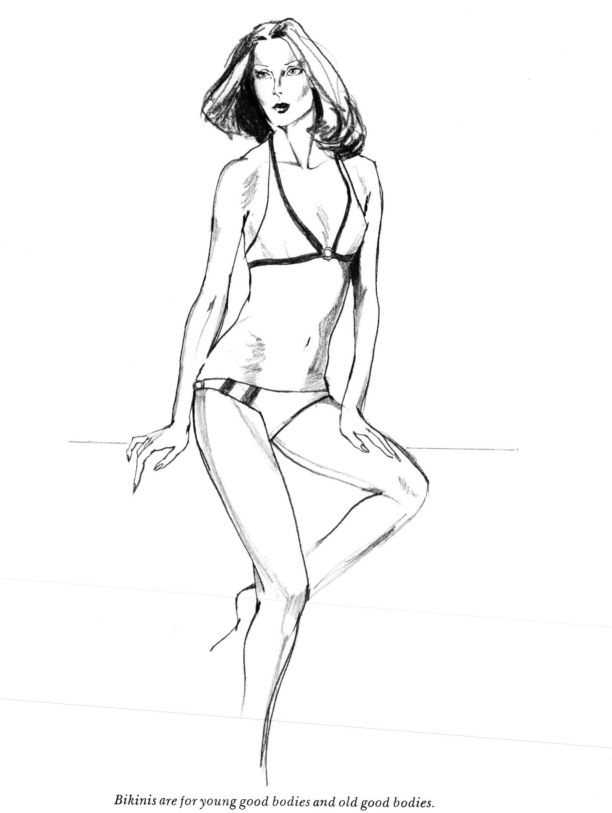

Bikinis are for young good bodies and old good bodies.

I feel a woman owes it to herself and to others at the beach not to offend them (or herself) by wearing something that makes her look gross. If you ask me who should wear bikinis, I'd say:

young, good bodies.

Or even:

old, good bodies.

If you're a sun-and-saltwater nut, I'd suggest finding a nudist beach and getting *all* of it. Or, if you don't have a good body and you insist on a bikini, try to keep to your end of the beach and wear a cover-up when you come to the snack bar to buy the hot dog you really don't need.

A word on bottomless and topless, the "monokini":

In my opinion, if you plan to go bottomless, it's better to just be nude. If you feel you have to cover your breasts, then keep your groin covered too. A woman with a top and no bottom simply looks scatter-brained and forgetful, and the garment that she *is* wearing is about as useful as a lid without anything to cover.

Topless is a different story. It's becoming more and more acceptable (in Europe more than in America), and we'll probably soon reach the point where breasts are no longer thought of as something that must be hidden from the public eye. Loose and sheer tops already reveal a lot of breasts. See-through blouses, if they're not too obvious, are acceptable even on Grace Kelly types. Going braless under knit and jersey tops means revealing the outline of the breasts and nipples. The actual topless surfaced for a short time in the sixties (through designer Rudi Gernreich), but though some women wore topless gowns in swinging London (that was the time of the Christine Keeler scandal), it never caught on (or off) here.

At that time I predicted—and my prediction still holds—that we'd be moving more and more toward breast exposure and might ultimately get back to the gowns worn first in Crete, then later in the Renaissance in Venice. The entire dress was designed then to push up and hold the exposed breasts high and round over a tight bodice.

We're definitely tending toward that. But whether you go topless or not will depend on where you are, and if you're willing to go along with it. I felt very uncomfortable at a topless beach in St. Tropez, though I eventually had to accept that when in Rome . . . and when in St. Tropez, too.

If you want to go topless, but don't want to stand out, you're most likely to blend in with the crowd on a French beach, whether in France itself or one of the French islands, like Martinique and Guadeloupe in the Caribbean. In St. Tropez anything *except* a topless is conspicuous and out of style.

Other countries with topless or nude beaches include Germany and Yugoslavia, Holland, Denmark and Jamaica. In Australia and Brazil, "the string" is popular—that little bit of twine taken from a crocheting basket to hold up three tiny patches. If you plan a nude, topless or string summer vacation, ask your travel agent or get in touch with the information services of the countries you're interested in and ask for names of beaches. Plan to leave out China and the Soviet Union on this particular trip.

Whatever you do or don't have on for swimming, you'll need additional beachwear for lounging, lunching and protection. The prettiest of all looks is an extremely large scarf in a marvelous print or dynamite color that will go with all your bathing suits. Sarong-tie this scarf around your hips or waist and you have a sensational, graceful outfit. Depending on the size of the scarf, it'll be a beautiful long or short skirt, with the bra or halter of your bathing suit on top. If you get a really super-sized scarf, you can tie it around your breasts and let it fall to the ground as a long summer dress.

These scarves will take you lots of places. They're extremely pretty, feminine, summery, and they conceal. To me, there's nothing quite so

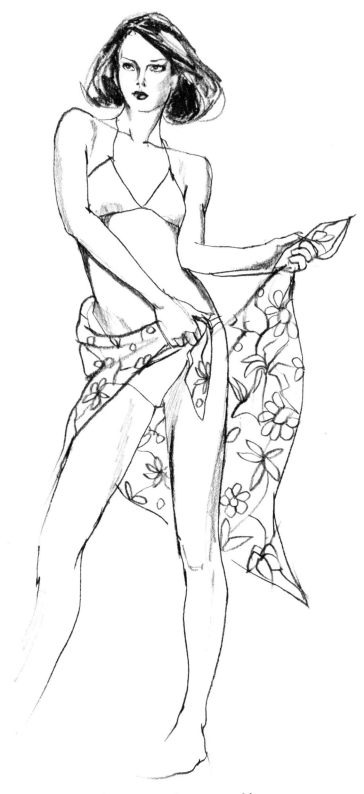

The super-size scarf can be a super skirt.

unattractive—usually—as the crotch of a bathing suit. Just to be able to cover that up and soften the line from waist or hips down is marvelous.

If you can't find the scarves, don't panic. I ran from store to store and could never find a really large scarf. Then I realized it wasn't a problem. I went into a fabric store, selected the fabric, had the square I wanted cut from it and didn't even have to bother sewing the edges because I had it cut with finishing scissors. At a fabric store or department, you have a much larger selection at much less cost than in the scarf section of a department store. And you can buy any size square you want.

These scarves are a particular joy to travelers. Pack three or four bathing suits and about eight scarves; they take up almost no room and you have an incredible variety of looks for day and even evening.

It's the most wonderful way in the world to dress. But you'll also need something to protect the upper part of your body. You'll need a beach wrap and a beach hat for protection. Most women don't realize how very dangerous the sun can be. Unless you have excessively oily skin, you shouldn't expose your face to the sun for longer than you have to. And take care of your body, too. Exposure to the sun should be very controlled, and you should never burn. It's not only dangerous; it's also uncomfortable and ugly. The most devastating evening dress won't draw attention away from raw, peeling skin.

The total beach wrap is an absolute *must*. I mean a garment or tops and bottoms that can protect *all* of you from the sun. Terry cloth is great fun and extremely practical. You don't have to get the old terry robe. New terries can be anything from very thin and clinging to thick, creamy plush with the look of velours, and they come in a great variety of styles. You can get a poncho, caftan, long T-shirt, sarong tie—or just a terry top to go with your large scarf. Terries are wonderful looking, a dream to care for and the most comfortable fabric in the world.

A beach hat is essential, even if you plan to wear kerchiefs. The

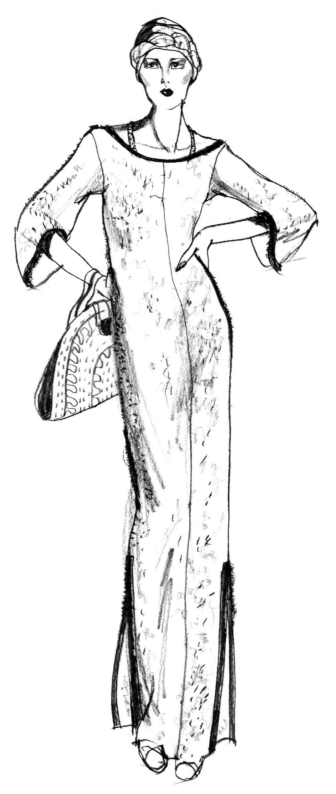

The total cover-up is an absolute must on the beach.

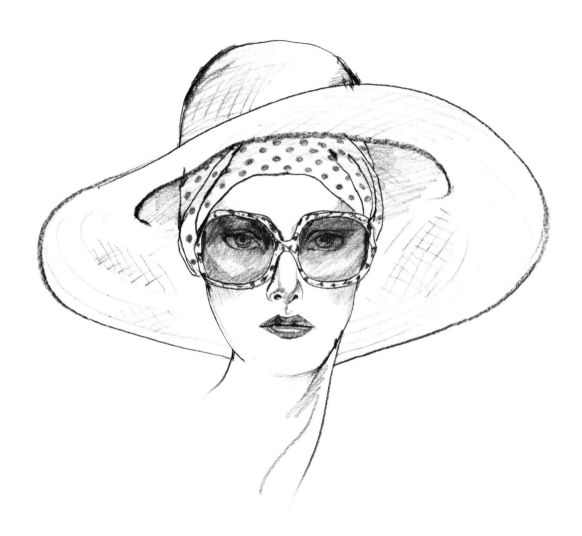

Beach chic.

kerchief protects your hair but not your face. You might need both, hat *and* scarf. When you come out of the water, you hair's soaking wet. Even if you wear a bathing cap, it's bound to be damp. You may be going directly from the beach to someone's house or to a restaurant for lunch and let's say you're not one of those lucky women who can just fluff dry their hair in the sun and look goregous. You tie your hair in the scarf and put the floppy straw hat on over it. The color of the scarf will show at the back of your head and maybe the sides. It's a very chic, put-together look that's also good for you.

I can't offer any suggestions about sunglasses, except try on at least a dozen. Choose the one that fits best on your head and suits the particular shape of your face. Be guided only by what's best on you and forget the oversized frames or granny glasses unless they really flatter you.

Now you're ready for the beach, from head to barefoot toe. It's wonderful, it feels free and natural to go barefoot all summer long—but it's not realistic. There will be times when you need shoes, if only for protection. Hot sand, rocky beaches, concrete and gravel are all very uncomfortable. And unless you're under eighteen and look it, don't try entering a restaurant without shoes.

For beachwear, a rubber-soled slipper is best. These slippers now come with a slightly wedged heel that will make your legs look more attractive than the flat thong sandal. A completely flat heel doesn't do much for your legs, and there are ways of wearing a heel without looking as though you are. The old look of Miss America in bathing suit and high heels sauntering down the runway at Atlantic City might be great if you're Miss America and on a runway, but it doesn't look good on a beach. Wedges and subtle heels are much more chic.

Above all, let your beachwear be totally washable. Anything that has to be dry-cleaned is no good for beach, lake or pool. If you're invited to jump in the pool after a black tie dinner when you're in your crepe de chine, my advice is either to decline the invitation or to throw all

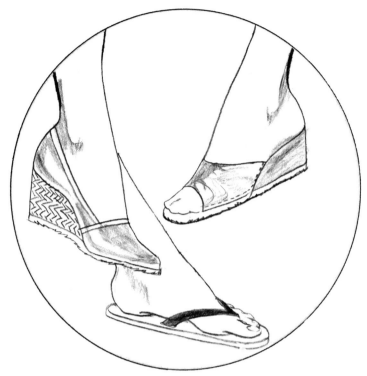

Make sure your beach slippers have rubber soles.

modesty to the winds. Better yet—don't throw. Hang the dress up carefully, far from the poolside, and ask your hostess for a towel.

Clear Sailing and Other Water Sports

For sailing, you'll need a couple of pairs of duck pants, sneakers or duck shoes, a windbreaker, shirts and a couple of turtleneck sweaters. Nights on the water are almost always bound to be cool. Take your bathing suit and *plenty* of moisturizer or sun creams. Whatever the sun can do to your skin on dry land, it does with double intensity on the water. Let your shirts double as cover-ups over your bathing suit. Work shirts and denim shirts look very nautical, particularly if you have a navy and white pirate-type kerchief over your hair.

For evening at the marina, take along dressy pants with a little top or halter. You can get tops that fold to the size of hankerchiefs or smaller—particularly those little wraparound tanks or halter-style tops. They're inexpensive and look great. You can dress them up with the right jewelry. They're also perfect if you decide to wear a long skirt, maybe an ankle-length (longer might be impractical) flowered skirt in a synthetic or any virtually wrinkle-proof material. A really great nautical-but-nice look at the discothèque is a pair of dazzling white, white pants with a bare halter. Get pants that are totally and unequivocally white, crisp, clean-looking and, of course, washable.

Bring your change of clothes along. They won't take up much room, they can hang out in the cabin, and you'll look much fresher in the evening than if you'd had them on all day.

If you're going out for serious water sports, you'll need specific equipment. But even regulation outfits can look fabulous if you get the right fit in the best color. The wet suits used for diving are among the sexiest items of apparel made. (Take the plunge and try them as costuming.) Whether short or full-length, they mold the body with sleekness and slickness, so if you're getting a wet suit for scuba diving, choose the one that's most knockout on land. It's a piece of equipment that can make the most of yours.

The same is true of life vests. If you're sailing with your favorite speed demon and don't know how to swim, get an all-in-one floatable in nylon or vinyl with little cap sleeves and a zipper up the front. It looks like a jump suit and keeps you safe. Even if you decide to wear a life vest only, there's no need for you to spend the day in a bulky, unattractive piece of equipment. You can find tested and secure life vests made of thin buoyant foam, and in many bright colors.

For serious swimming and water-skiing, get a *swimming* swimming suit. I mean one that's sturdy, with bottoms that stay up and straps that stay put. Make especially sure that your bottoms fit snugly at the waist or hips—or else you may take a beautiful dive and realize when you're coming up that your pants are twenty feet below you. I know from experience. I've started off on water skis, taken a spill and, as I was coming up out of the water, realized my pants wanted to stay at water level. That realization is enough to make you lose your composure. You find yourself holding on to your bottoms with one hand and the bar with the other.

If a bathing cap is part of your equipment, you don't have to be too serious about it—unless you plan to swim the Channel or across Lake Michigan. (If so, consult a more professional guide than this on what to wear for the marathon.) I find there's not too much difference in the water-tightness of caps. None of them really keeps the water out completely. So instead of wearing the standard white cap that makes you look as though you've just had surgery, buy any of the new amusing kinds. Get one that looks like a wig, and be a redhead or a platinum blonde or whatever mermaid-self you fantasize. Your hair won't be dry when you come out of the water, but it won't be soaking wet either.

I always take hot curlers along when I'm going somewhere for real swimming. They let me do a quick touch-up in the evening, and by day I wear a kerchief or hat or both if my hair is damp.

Whenever you go out on or into the water, take along a cover-up. Take two: a light one for protection against sun rays and a warmer one against wind or chill. If you can go without makeup, you're a step ahead of the game. If you feel you really need it, use as little as possible (bright eye shadow on the water looks simply silly) and get the most waterproof products you can find. Esther Williams may have come up from the briny deeps with absolutely perfect makeup in her movies, but don't forget there were a lot of people around to help her. When you're coming out of the pool, you can't shout, "Cut!", and if your mascara is down at your jaw line, people may think you're starting to melt.

Roughing It

There are standard items I take and have always taken for camping trips: blue jeans, of course, and corduroys, halter tops, peasant blouses (lots of overblouses), turtleneck sweaters (many), sweater sets and, to pack it all in, either a windbreaker, a fun fur or a leather jacket.

Camping covers a host of ills—and delights. It's everything from a rough two weeks' hike in mountainous terrain with a heavy rucksack to a deluxe trailer. For the rougher versions, I'd suggest forgetting about evening wear and frilly night clothes. If you'll be sleeping in a tent, don't take your negligee, even if it's a pup tent sized for one and a half people and the other occupant is Robert Redford. I'd still take comfortable pajamas—great-looking, man-tailored, in washable cotton. They should be slightly large on you; a woman looks *very* provocative in a man's oversized pajama top.

If you'll be spending the night in a sleeping bag, even if you're sharing it, again I suggest you leave your sheer black gown at home. Comfortable pajamas in this situation will do the trick. If it's cold enough, you won't even change out of your jeans or hiking pants. This is one time when a bird (or man) in hand is the only one you can get, and if you're sharing a sleeping bag he'd be an idiot to prowl, so forget about the come-hither clothes and concentrate on creature comforts.

If, however, you're traveling in a camper, there's nothing wrong with packing one negligee. A negligee in the wilderness can be extremely effective, and it's also convenient in the morning, when you're eating your peeled grapes under the canopy within eyeshot of fellow campers.

For daytime, jeans are perfect. Hiking is what jeans were invented for. If it's hot and you want to wear shorts, don't. Not if they're short shorts, that is. Your legs will be unprotected and you'll have to pick your way branch by branch and thorn by thorn. If you really hate the warmth of long pants, compromise with Bermuda shorts and wear knee-high socks.

Pack a few scarves in your rucksack and take hot rollers along in your camper. Make sure you have enough body lotion, cleanser, rinser and whatever other cosmetics you need for the trip. It's a good idea to to take moisturizer with a sun-screen ingredient if you'll be out in the sun a lot. And if you plan to get tanned on this trip, take a darker makeup along in addition to your regular makeup, to use when the tan starts coming through. If you'll be in a sunny place, take bright lipsticks and bright eye shadows. (But save them for evening; it's gauche to plod the woodland paths with violet lids.)

A marvelous item for camping trips is the travel wig. It doesn't have to be set, is synthetic and can always be rinsed out. It's just as good for long boating trips. If you've spent a long, hot, exhausting day on the yacht, have come home before going out to the Winter Casino in Monte Carlo to do a little gambling, and have no time for the beauty salon or even to set your hair, this is really the answer. Even in the Everglades or Yosemite Park, a cute, contemporary wig can take you from sporty day to glamorous night in seconds. As far as I'm concerned, it's tops.

Oh Say, Can You Ski?

Even if you can't, you can look as though you're ready for the giant slalom. Skiing is always an investment, and you might as well start out on the right two feet. Look as streamlined and nifty as possible on the slopes, with the sleekest (though still comfortable) pants, parka and sweaters around. If you're only there for the après ski, stay in bed all day or consult with the hotel chef, but don't venture on the mountain in ski-bunny clothes. You might be so cute that nobody notices you don't have a cottontail, but serious skiers and ski teachers are not going to stop in midschuss to help you with your bindings or find your mittens.

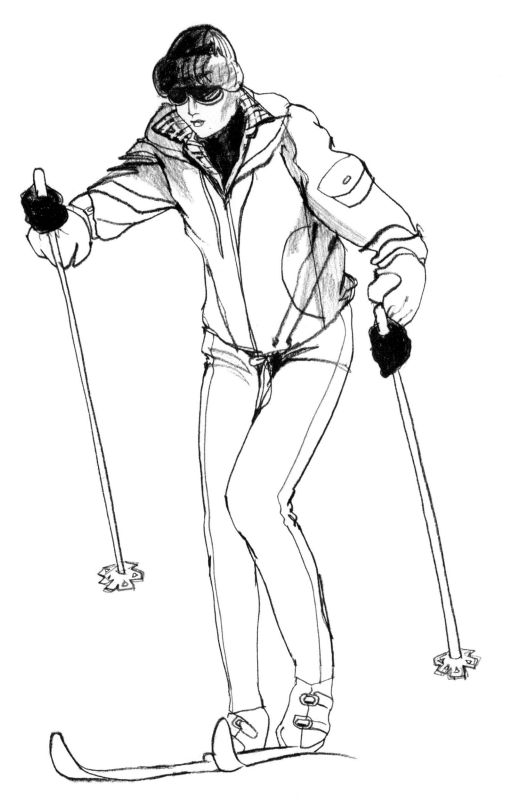

Look as streamlined and nifty as possible.

The sensational gold jump suit is fine after dark; on the slopes it's an eyesore. If you plan on skiing, get the equipment you need for the sport. That means boots, first of all (you can rent skis and poles, but your own boots are the first investment you should make). Not too long ago, new ski boots were a minor form of hell-on-earth, the masochist's delight. They blistered and bruised on the long tortuous way to proper fit, and the greatest moment of the ski day came when you returned from the slopes in the afternoon, took off the boots and soaked your poor feet. Wealthy customers in the Alps would ask ski teachers to break in their boots for them over the summer.

It also took forever to get into them, with their double sets of laces, inside and out. They usually had to be tightened again after an hour's skiing. This alone insured that only those who cared about skiing were on the slopes.

Now boots are buckled, often foam-filled and wearable even when new. Since you ski with your feet more than with any other part of the body, your boots are the most important part of all your skiing equipment. They're expensive, but should last more or less forever. That's one reason to get them in a color that will go with all the different ski pants and skis you will own over the years. If you choose a brilliant color for your boots, you'll be limited in choice for the rest of your outfit.

Give yourself plenty of time for trying on boots. Test them in the shop by doing ski movements. Put all your weight forward, then back, then distribute it evenly. Move your feet from side to side as though you were turning. The boot should hold you, keeping your heel down, but it shouldn't cut into you. You should be able to wiggle your toes. Pay attention to the necessary space at the top of the boot.

You need ski pants or overalls, long underwear, parka or windbreaker, ski gloves (or mittens), goggles, warm socks and cap. Each part of this equipment is necessary and useful. Ski pants are waterproof, stream-lined and held down at the feet. No other pants give you those ad-

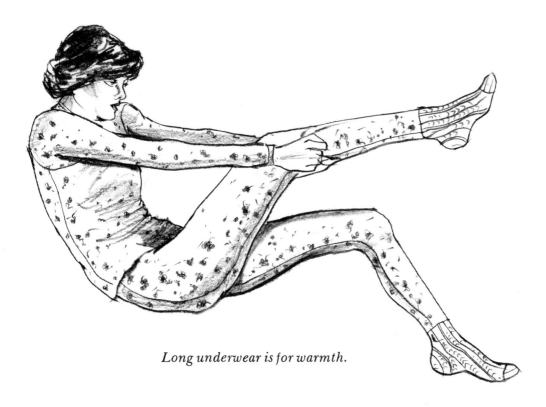

Long underwear is for warmth.

vantages, and jeans should be worn for skiing only as the last resort. Long underwear is for warmth, and you'll need it. Cotton or thermal long johns can be very pretty in a garden color or print. You can substitute tights if you wish, but they probably won't give you the warmth or comfort you'll need.

Your jacket will depend on where and when you ski. Down parkas, even in the coldest weather, have the disadvantage of being bulky and not easy to maneuver in. You might need one for really icy weather, but I'd recommend building up warmth through layers under a thinner parka over it. You'll need the jacket even for spring or summer skiing, though for very hot weather (glacier skiing in summer), a thin nylon shell is enough. You need the jacket to keep you dry in spills and to keep you warm going up on the lift.

181

Never ski without gloves, even in the hottest weather, or you'll chap and break your skin. If you're wearing sunglasses instead of (or in addition to) goggles, make sure the lenses are impact-resistant.

Choose a cap that will keep your ears warm, your hair in place and will stay on your head. You don't want to sift through mountains of snow after a fall trying to find it.

All this equipment can be very chic and colorful. Most people look tremendous in a ski outfit. It's the long, lean look from head to toe, and can be made to look longer and leaner if you wear one color from top to bottom.

You should be able to peel layers when the day gets warmer or when you come into the hut for a hot chocolate. Start your layering with a thin sweater or long-sleeved T-shirt. Wear a shirt over that, tucked into your ski pants. That's all you'll need in the hut, and it'll look fabulous. Ski pants are the most perfect garment for women who are slightly overweight. They mold and control, slimming down the body from waist to ankles.

Over the shirt, wear a sweater that's not tucked in (if you can tuck in the sweater comfortably, your pants are probably too loose), then your parka or windbreaker over the sweater. Make sure the colors you wear match each other or are coordinated. There's no reason why you shouldn't look like oiled lightning. Base your outfit on whatever color suits you best, and if you're overweight try to stay with darker colors.

The reflection of the sun against the snow is very strong. No matter how oily your skin, you'll need protection. Use sun screens. Get the sun products made specially for skiers, and reapply them often. If lipstick isn't enough to protect your lips, use a cream or ointment made to prevent skin chapping or breaking. Never forget the sun. At the beach, you can wear a hat. On the slopes, you rely completely on lotions, creams and oils.

For après-ski, again the first thing you need are boots. Fur ones are fun and attractive and serve the purpose of keeping the snow out.

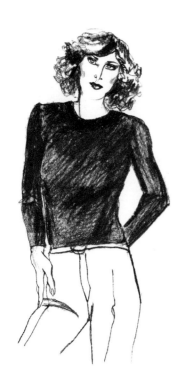

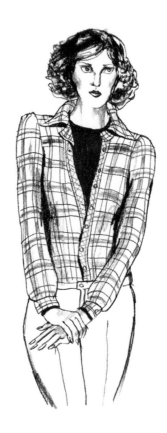

Add layers for more warmth.

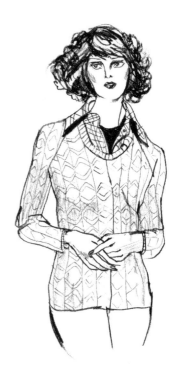

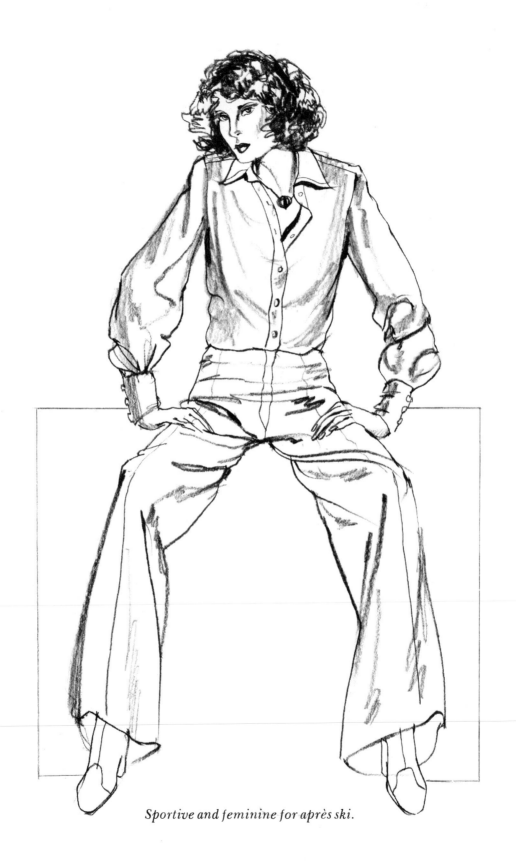

Sportive and feminine for après ski.

Your boots should let you walk through the snow to the discothèque without getting your feet wet and should be comfortable enough to dance in when you get there.

Unless you're going to an ultra-elegant ski resort, you won't need any formal evening wear. One long skirt or long wool (or cashmere) dress is ample for just-in-case. Otherwise, take your favorite pants and tops. If you love jeans and look good in them, you can get by in most places. But let at least one pair be velvet or velveteen. If you have dressy pants, lounging pajamas, jump suits, take them. In most places you can go wearing anything from jeans to a long dress and look right in all outfits. (We'll talk about the more elegant European ski resorts in the next chapter.)

Don't clutter your luggage with evening clothes you can wear only once. A pair of well-fitting jeans with a white silk shirt is super, and you can dress it up with jewelry, belt, scarf or—if you're going braless—unbutton it as far as you dare.

Other Winter Sports

You have more leeway in dressing for the other sports. Except for specific equipment—skates, snowshoes, sleds—you can be guided by your need for warmth, comfort and maneuverability. If you're skating indoors, you can wear the classic Sonja Henie skating outfit with the little round skirt and flesh-colored tights. But you can also go in jeans and a sweater, if the jeans are tight and held in your boots.

For tobogganing, bobsledding and old-fashioned sleigh rides, bundle up and wear an adorable cap or hat. Find a brightly colored wool scarf to wrap around your neck, and keep your feet warm, your hair dry and your skin moist. Take along a thermos of something hot or a flask of something strong.

6

Roaming

April in Paris

Chestnuts in blossom. The Seine, mistress of Paris, rolling by, lovers strolling along her banks. Josephine Baker used to sing, "J'ai deux amours—mon pays et Paris." In the mid-twenties it was said that good Americans go to Paris when they die, and later Gene Kelly, in *An American in Paris*, kept alive the belief that Paris was as close to Paradise as we could reasonably expect to get.

Americans have loved Paris for a long time and have loved all of her: sidewalk cafés, the Folies Bergères, Montmartre, the Champs-Élysées, Notre Dame on the Ile de la Cité, the Eiffel Tower at Trocadero, the wine, the smells, elegance, fashion, romance—the promise of everything and anything. Of all cities, Paris is the most evocative, sensual and creative.

You're winging your way to Paris in springtime, sampling a little Beaujolais on the plane with your pâté. Your baggage is in the hold. Your coat, your camera and umbrella are in the baggage rack. Your handbag is at your side and your carry-on bag is at your feet. You dread the landing, when you'll have to gather up everything and stagger down the aisle, as you staggered up through it when you boarded.

Roaming

At this point in your life, you're grateful you don't have a baby. There was a young family at your check-in counter with carrying crib, stroller, stuffed animals, baby bottles, baby food and packages of paper diapers. On another line, a businessman was carrying trench coat, briefcase, camera, tape recorder, umbrella and typewriter. An elegant woman in a tailored suit held only a beautiful leather carryall. How was she going to find her passport in it, and wouldn't she freeze on those "sometimes-the-air-is-surprisingly-fresh" evenings the travel agent told you about?

I've never discovered how to board a plane without looking like a native bearer on a safari. The forty-four pounds you're allowed in economy (sixty-six pounds, first class) can definitely be worked out with a little planning. But that still leaves the breakables (camera, typewriter, tape recorder), the unpackables (umbrellas, hats, fur coat) and the items needed on flight (toiletries, brush and comb, books). You have to be careful, though, not to be obvious about carrying too much or your hand luggage might be weighed.

I always pack cosmetics and toiletries in a separate bag that I carry on the plane. I advise everyone to do so. The way luggage is handled, you have a good chance of even plastic bottles and jars spilling or bursting. Also, you'll want your makeup at hand so you can freshen up before you land. Unless you plan on carrying a small bag designed exclusively for cosmetics, it's most practical to get one, two or as many cosmetics bags as you need and pack all your grooming items into them before putting the bags in whatever case you bring aboard. These cosmetics bags have waterproof linings (in case anything leaks), and many have compartments where you can neatly pack small items like hairpins or eye shadows.

Take along everything you normally need for grooming—your moisturizers, body lotions, night creams, cleansers, rinsers, hair products and makeup. If your hair is bleached or dyed, take along a color rinse that will cover the roots and let you go for a longer time between touch-ups. It's also a good idea to get the formula for your color from your colorist. Many products are the same in Europe or have equivalents that would be recognized in a good European salon.

If you're going abroad for a long time, don't feel you have to carry a total supply of everything. Most products sold in America are also sold in Europe and you can probably find your favorite brands. If not, the European equivalent might be just as good or better. The only exception to this would be if you have hyper-allergic skin and need very special preparations. In that case, you probably can't afford to gamble on finding them abroad.

Don't take along a traveling hospital either, even if you're traveling with children. Band-Aids and aspirins, rubbing alcohol, iodine and all other first-aid items are available in any pharmacy. So are toothpaste, shampoo, mouthwash, soaps and anything else you need for cleanliness. So take the products you normally use in a quantity convenient for packing. If you use a well-known fragrance, you can probably buy it duty-free at the airport in cologne, perfume or talc form.

Because you'll be packing a color-coordinated wardrobe (I'll tell you about that in a minute), you won't need a wardrobe of makeup colors. I used to take a ton of makeup. I don't anymore. Coordinating the colors of my clothes means coordinating the colors of my makeup.

When you start planning what to take, think of the color you like best or have the most of. Make that the basis of your wardrobe and coordinate bulky, essential items (like shoes and bags) with it. You're best off if you select a neutral color as your base. The earth colors are good, particularly beige. (I'm basing my travel wardrobe on beige this year.) Black, white or black and white are also excellent.

This doesn't mean you have to be monotonous or monochrome. You can still take that one powerhouse fuchsia dress, or the knock-'em-dead lounging pajamas in Chinese red. Just don't forget you'll need shoes, a bag, accessories and makeup to go with it.

If you base your wardrobe on a single color, you can have a tremendous variety of outfits with a minimal number of garments. Your bags and shoes will go with everything you have. So will your coat or jacket. If you pack a café au lait skirt, beige pants and a chocolate brown jacket, you can then brighten up or tone down the outfit as much as you please. A matching silk shirt with the café au lait skirt is very ladylike. But you can also wear a bright tunic or a vibrant sweater.

I experiment with color through accessories. If there's a new color of the season, I don't buy a complete outfit in it. I'll get a scarf or belt first and see whether the color suits me or not. Most women know what color they look best in, but it's good to experiment. Often you're happily surprised, and wearing some color for the first time can make a woman feel adventurous or new.

When you're traveling, take accessories in any color you like, but economize on space and weight by packing standard and essential items that are all color-coordinated. You'll save time and headaches throughout your trip. If everything in your hotel closet is color-coordinated, you won't have to go through agonies trying to figure out what to wear every day.

Also, decide which items of jewelry match your outfits, and make your decisions before you go. Jewelry can take up a lot of room. Pack only what you need for the outfits you take.

Take synthetics, knits and wash-and-wear. Leave anything that needs dry cleaning at home. You may not be in any one place long enough to send things out to the cleaners, and you won't want to waste space by traveling around the Continent with a suitcase full of dirty clothes.

The garments you pack should also hang out easily. Even if you take a travel iron with you—a good idea, incidentally, for touch-ups—you may not have the space or time to iron everything out. Besides, it's a chore and a bore. Take clothes that will look fresh if they're hung up or lightly steamed in the bathroom while you're taking a shower.

Lightweight knits are marvelous. You can take knit pants and roll them—literally roll them—in a tight ball and stick them around the sides of your luggage. They unroll when you hang them up and an hour later you have them on. The same goes for knit tops, jackets and skirts. All of these come in summery fabrics and colors and are great for daytime or evening.

The travel iron is good for touching up collars and other spot ironing. A steam iron is best, and make sure you have an adapter along for European current. It's more economical to take an adapter than to buy an iron specifically made for use in Europe. You may have other electrical items with you—like an electric toothbrush, razor, hot rollers, hair dryer—and the adapter will fit all of them.

Choose things that don't wrinkle, but pack as though they did, for extra insurance. Your suitcase should be large enough to hold all forty-four pounds. Each item of baggage weighs something by itself, and it's more fun to take a few extra tops and scarves than to have to limit yourself because you're traveling with a few pieces of luggage. Also, you may find yourself in airports or train stations at night with no porter to help. Try never to take more luggage than you could handle by yourself, if you had to.

Buy the lightest luggage available. I once received a set of beautiful Vuitton luggage from my husband as a Christmas present. It was sensational, the most gorgeous luggage I've ever seen. But *empty*, it used up most of the baggage weight allowance.

So get lightweight luggage, but make sure it isn't so flimsy that it falls apart before you're in the air. The more support it gives, the better your clothes will be held in place and the fresher they'll look when you unpack. I don't believe in investing a lot of money in a suitcase. Even expensive luggage is liable to arrive at its destination with the handles ripped off or the zipper torn. Most travelers have had the experience of watching their luggage come down the ramp with half its contents sticking out and maybe a cord tied around it—if they're lucky. If you travel a lot, don't count on keeping your luggage too long, no matter how fine its quality.

A large, sturdy, lightweight suitcase with some frame to it is best. You must be able to lock it, and if you have a tendency to lose keys, buy a combination lock and set it to numbers that you won't forget. Your birthdate, anniversary or some other important date in your life is less forgettable than random numbers. Your suitcase should have straps on the inside to hold everything securely in place. If the straps are missing, use ribbons or soft belts from your robe or raincoat.

Lay down the belts first, or make sure the luggage straps are out so you don't find yourself at the end all neatly packed and the straps lost somewhere in the middle. Now bring on the heaviest items—shoes, bags, books. Use the space in your bags for hose and panties or jewelry if you're not taking a special jewelry case. The best jewelry cases are made of a soft fabric, like suede, and can be rolled up and tied. There's never enough room in them, though, so you might have to resort to using the side pockets of the suitcase in addition.

Place small, soft items between the hard ones. Stockings can go into the toes of your shoes. Pack across, making one smooth level before you go on to the next. The basic principle of packing is to have heavier things on the bottom, lighter things on top, with everything *packed in* so it doesn't move around. Leather belts go around the sides of the suitcase at the base. Sweaters and jeans should be packed before dresses.

If you have the patience, lay tissue paper in the folds when you're folding your skirts and dresses. This reduces wrinkles. Keep your long skirts and dresses for the end and finish off the job with your robe as a sort of cover for all the contents. Don't pack so full that you couldn't possibly squeeze another thing in. No matter where you're going, you're bound to buy *something*, and you'll need room to bring it back in. Strap everything in, zip the bag up, lock the lock and attach baggage tags. They should be filled out with your home and foreign addresses. Luggage is lost more often than airline companies like to admit, and your chances of ever getting it back are severely diminished if there's no address on it.

For April in Paris, you'll need the same basic suits, dresses, skirts or pants you'd wear in an American city. The only important difference is that Europeans don't overheat their rooms, and if you're used to wearing your bare halter dress to cocktail parties at eighty-degree temperatures, you'll definitely be chilly in Paris. Unless the weather really turns freakish, you won't need anything sleeveless or bare.

Most French women dress with a lot of chic. The French are body-conscious, and French clothes are body-revealing on both men and women. French men wore very tight, form-fitting trousers years ago, when American men still favored loose-to-baggy pants.

In spite of the fame of Paris fashions, the French now dress in the casual sporty look developed by American designers. They love jeans and T-shirts and simple lines. And perfect fit always. No matter how casually she dresses, be she salesgirl or countess, the French woman is always *chic*. When she takes over "le T-shirt"—whether it's long- or short-sleeved; V-necked, boat-necked or crew-necked; to the hips, the knees or the floor—it gently molds the body and leaves you in no doubt as to what she has on or has left off underneath.

The French led fashion for centuries, when all clothes were custom-made. In an age of ready-made dressing, they still haven't lost their flair. Details are extremely important to them, as is the quality of the material. A French woman can take the simplest dress, or a plain navy skirt and white top, and with a scarf, a brooch and a belt turn it into an outfit with all the élan of high fashion.

The French dress the way they cook, taking a little something, adding a pinch of this, a soupçon of that and ending up with some magnificent concoction. Like most European women, the French buy garments to keep for many years, preferring the one really good suit to three or four inexpensive ones which might have to be replaced in a year or two. A woman with a low income will save up for that magnificent all-silk scarf (Hermès?) instead of buying a few in rayon.

Don't try to look French in France. You won't succeed unless you look French to begin with. Wherever you are, wear the clothes you're accustomed to and are comfortable with. You don't change your personality with each new country you visit, and there's no reason to change your wardrobe either. A good rule to go by is: Dress in anything you'd put on for a similar occasion at home *unless* you know that this would be offensive or misunderstood. For example, you might wear a pants suit to church at home, but in some Latin countries pants are still considered disrespectful.

What you specifically pack for Paris depends on where and for how long you'll be staying, and what you're likely to be doing. The Right Bank of Paris is more formal than the Left. If you're staying in one of the really elegant Paris hotels—the George V, Ritz, Crillon—then you'll probably also be dining at Tour d'Argent, Maxim's or Lapérouse. Take your most elegant dinner clothes or cocktail dresses, and be sure to include some long evening dresses.

For the Left Bank, you'll want more casual clothes. Jeans are fine for strolling along St. Germain or the Boul' Mich'. Little theaters and clubs won't require formal clothes, and you might feel like sitting on the banks of the Seine or picnicking in the Luxembourg Gardens.

With worldwide inflation, you won't find bargains in most European countries. Paris on the whole is shockingly expensive. But if you want to pick up an extra something, to have your own little piece of Parisian chic, try Galeries Lafayette or Bon Marché, two large department stores that have just about everything at the most reasonable prices you can expect.

Plan to spend most of your money on food. Dining in Paris is always an exciting adventure, even in little out-of-the-way places on the Left Bank. French people honor food, so don't be surprised if the ladies are in silk dresses with pearls even in a small restaurant. If the food is very good, customers pay their compliments to the chef by dressing as though the occasion were important.

When in Paris, eat, drink and fall in love. Even if the effects of all three have gone by morning, your memories will still be fresh when you return home.

London at Any Season

It will almost certainly be chilly. Many of the English still look on central heating as something unhealthy or too pampering or whatever. Puritan forebears considered wrong whatever gave pleasure or comfort, and this streak, though dying out finally, still lingers on in England. It accounts for cold rooms and overcooked food. If you'll be traveling through the countryside at any season—even summer—be sure to take some warm clothes along. "Woolies" is a term of endearment used by the English to describe those garments that make life tolerable.

There's another side to England too, of course, and it's getting stronger all the time. England swings. Before the sixties, when the Queen's designer was Hartnell, English ladies were stout, sensible (at best "handsome") and dowdy in their dress. When the sixties brought a revolution in lifestyle and clothing, little shops opened in Chelsea and Soho, with mod, mad clothes. Vidal Sassoon's first salon, on Bond Street, introduced the concept of using scissors instead of rollers, cutting hair to suit the woman's facial structure and cutting *into* the curl so the hair would keep its shape. New, sometimes crazy makeup was developed and worn with obvious artifice. Girls, and later boys, blossomed in new colors and new styles. Swinging London became the mod capital of the world; minis were micro, bras were left off and there was such a general joy in dressing that at times it felt like a carnival.

There's no line to tread between the two extremes. The conservative

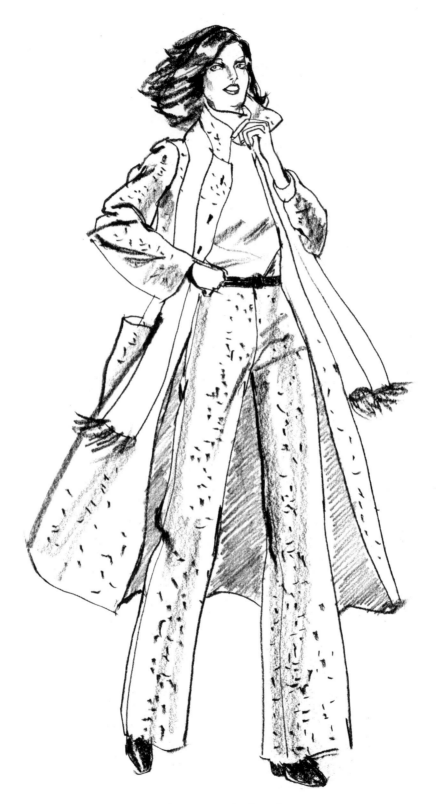

Stay warm in London.

dressers haven't changed. You can still find the old-fashioned English-man who trusts his tailor more than his wife or the prime minister. As he hails a cab in homburg and umbrella, out flies the typical English bird, dressed in jeans or a long skirt, or any kind of costume at all. She looks as though she never actually *decided* what to wear; these clothes were simply at hand and she put them on.

In London, anything goes most any place you're going. Again, wear the same clothes you'd wear back home, with the precaution of bringing along an additional sweater or jacket. Though most public places are now heated, they're often not heated adequately by American standards so London, despite its moderate climate, is one of the coldest cities of Western Europe.

If you own any outfit you love but can never wear because it's always too hot due to indoor heating in winter, and outdoor heat in summer, definitely take it along to England. You can wear thick wools and tweeds, angoras and cashmeres without feeling you're in a Turkish bath. Of course, it does get warm in summer, and can even be very hot, so don't cover yourself from head to toe in the thermal clothes if you're going in August. But *do* take a suit or dress with jacket, and a few extra cover-ups.

London is generally informal. It's a very private city, and much of the social life of London takes place at home. The theater is *not* an occasion for fancy dress, unless you're going to a command performance. Otherwise, you can wear anything from pants to knit suit or very underplayed dinner dress. In London's theaters, as on Broadway, you can tell the provincials because they're more dressed up than the native city folk. Most restaurants and informal clubs are casual. A pair of velvet pants with a soft blouse or silk shirt will be appropriate for everything but the grandest eating places.

There are a few black tie occasions in London—going to the private gambling clubs or charity balls, presentation to the Queen—but unless there's a strong chance you'll be in such a situation, don't bother packing your grand evening clothes. At the Savoy or Mirabelle's, in discothèques or for dinner-dancing, you'll never need anything more formal than your shocking pink silk lounging pajamas. You can dress as extravagantly as you wish (except for obvious, serious grand galas) in London and, as long as you don't disturb the horses, nobody will lift an eyelid.

If you're watching the races at Epsom Downs, you can wear your favorite My Fair Lady dress, complete with gloves and wide-brimmed hat, or you can dress fancifully. Ascot always produces strange costumes. One year a woman came in an outfit of fresh daisies sewn onto a net backing. She kept the dress in the refrigerator overnight and appeared at the racetrack looking delightfully crisp and cool.

You may not want to go as far as that. Also, you might catch cold. Whether you dress as a forest sprite or as Liza Doolittle, don't forget your cardigan.

If you don't have enough sweaters before leaving for England, try to wait until you get there. English woolens remain a joy. You can go to Harrods in Knightsbridge, the world's most complete department store, which sells everything from American breakfast foods to elephants.

There, you can find the classic tailored wool suit or go upstairs to the mirror-plated, rock-playing floor for kinky little outfits.

Harrods has wonderful garments of the highest quality, but is expensive. Selfridges on Oxford Street is a less expensive version of the store, though you won't be able to purchase elephants there.

But the best buys in London are at Marks and Spencer, a chain of low-price stores specializing in sweaters of all styles and knits. The chain is affectionately known as "Marks and Sparks" and should be a must on your list if you're planning to shop for yourself or for gifts to bring back home. They have many other items besides sweaters, and most Englishwomen—whether debs, journalists, actresses, secretaries or housewives—will check in from time to time.

If you're going to an English country house for the weekend, take your woolies and sensible walking shoes. Whenever you leave the city, take shoes you can walk in comfortably. The English expect to walk, even in a drizzle, and you won't want to miss the beautiful green English countryside because your feet hurt. This is especially true if you're going up north to the highlands. Instead of walking on paths, you'll probably go through fields and along riverbeds.

Wherever you go in England, remember that the climate can be very changeable. Spring can come in February and you can get chilled in September. Days are often misty or foggy, and it's extremely rare that a day is bright, clear and sunny from sunrise to sunset. You'll definitely need rainwear and shoes that keep you dry. If you're taking a winter coat, make sure that rain can't hurt it.

The moistness of English weather has been held responsible for giving Englishwomen the best complexions in the world. Let your skin breathe the benefits. If you have to wear makeup, make it light and porous. And, because the climate itself will often keep you dewy and moist, wear waterproof products on your eyes.

You'll find that in many parts of England the water is incredibly soft. Soap lathers into a froth on your skin. Take advantage of this water and, even if you're accustomed to showers at home, luxuriate in a long, warm bath.

Dr. Johnson said, "There is in London all that life can afford." That was in the eighteenth century, though it's probably still true today. London is an enormous, sprawling city, and each part of it has a different mood. Try to get up and out after early morning tea. Take your raincoat, put on comfortable shoes and explore Europe's largest metropolis from the Tower of London to Trafalgar Square, from St. Paul's Cathedral to Westminster Abbey; then come back for tea, take off your shoes, sink into a bath and get ready for what is probably the finest theater in the world.

Winter Vacations

When I'm flying over for a ski vacation in Switzerland, I put all my ski clothes (the two pairs of ski pants, the two jackets and my sweaters) in the duffel bag I carry on the plane with me. Though I'm not a professional weight lifter, I can handle it easily, balancing myself with a large handbag, almost the size of the duffel bag, in my other hand.

This leaves my suitcase free for everything else. Mainly, it gives me room to pack my boots. Now, ordinarily, I'll never pack boots; they're heavy and take up an enormous amount of room. But when I'm going skiing, boots are almost the only thing I pack, and I pack two pairs—one for day, the other for evening. I'll also put in some long T-shirt dresses, tops, pants, night clothes and underwear—but the suitcase is basically filled with boots.

You don't need many clothes on a ski vacation. Whether it's Gstaad, Switzerland, Aspen, Vail or Kitzbühel, Austria, you're headed for, there's no point packing anything dressy because you simply will never wear it. In Gstaad, I stayed at the Palace Hotel, where it might have been possible to put on a black tie outfit for the discothèque downstairs. But I just wore the long cashmere T-shirt dresses that I'd rolled up in my suitcase, and I was certainly dressy enough.

Fun T-shirts are great to have for ski evenings—the long-sleeved ones in a knit with decorations on them; words, pictures or tuxedo top printed on.

If you're planning a ski vacation in Europe and you don't know the place, you might ask your travel agent or the national tourist bureau about types of dress worn there—just in case. There *are* a few dressy places where you might feel a little awkward in pants, or where you'd regret the missed opportunity for dressing up. Ski resorts that cater to royalty will generally offer an excuse for black tie. The Palace Hotel in St. Moritz is quite formal. So is the Zürser Hof in Zürs (Austria).

Though that hotel has given up its practice of requiring black tie dress Monday evenings, it still numbers among its clients monarchs and potentates with entourage and dressy clothes.

Sometimes you have a choice. The younger people in the hotel will generally dress more informally and the older women will wear long dresses or long skirts. Sometimes the distinctions are not between generations but nationalities, and Americans tend to dress more informally than many Europeans.

If you'll be at the ski resort over New Year's, take a wonderful long dress or gown for New Year's Eve. It doesn't have to be brocade (though if that's what you want to wear, take it); it can be a simple wool or synthetic. Also, Christmas Eve is celebrated all over Europe. Take something long and elegant (though not formal) for the occasion. You won't need anything special for Christmas Day—everybody will be out on the slopes in their ski pants.

The key word for daily dressing at practically all ski resorts is "sporty." It can be sporty-chic or sporty-fun, but the mood of the day is somehow carried into the evening. If you intend to combine your ski vacation with other traveling involving business or pleasure, you have a nice little problem on your hands as far as packing goes.

Everything you need for the ski vacation will fit comfortably within the forty-four-pound limit. Skis, poles and boots are not part of the baggage allowance. Put the boots into the bindings, tie skis and poles securely and send them as a separate package for a nominal fee. Your two weeks in St. Moritz or Kitzbühel are now perfectly provided for.

But you have business in Zurich or Munich, and you want to stop over in Brussels for a few days before going home. You don't want to arrive in each city with skis and boots and luggage full of ski clothes. Nothing at all that you'd take to St. Moritz is appropriate for your meeting in Zurich or your lunch in Munich.

My first reaction to such a problem is that it shouldn't exist. It's impossible. There's no way on earth to pack for the Alps and the cities in one suitcase. Better to come home, unpack and start all over again. But I realize this may be impractical for some people. They're taking their ski vacation abroad precisely because they have to be there anyway and the fare is already taken care of.

One thing is inevitable: You will *have* to pay extra for luggage. This doesn't mean you have to pay the rate for overweight. Go to the airport early, or the day before if you can, and send a suitcase by air freight as unaccompanied baggage. Pack whatever you'll need for your city traveling, send it to the airport where you'll first be arriving, and when you get there, pick it up and check it. Now go off for your two weeks' skiing. When you return to the airport, send off your ski luggage and pick up your city luggage. It's not cheap, but it's more economical and less of a burden than carrying all your luggage with you all the time.

Of course there *are* people who can do all in one. There are also people who can build cars from scratch, speak twenty languages or calculate the distances between stars. I'm not one of them. To me, a business trip and a skiing vacation require two different wardrobes. But if you want to take a chance on packing it all together, start off with ski pants cut to look like regular pants, with a straight leg coming over the boots. Take only one pair of boots (you'll need room for shoes), wear a suit with skirt on the plane and coordinate your city clothes with the precision of a watchmaker. You'll have no more than fifteen pounds for all your city wear, so make sure every single item— every scarf, every piece of jewelry, every pair of stockings—will go with everything else you have.

If you're tempted to splurge on overweight and take whatever you want, never mind the cost—don't. Even if the money means nothing to you, the hassle of carting around lots of luggage can ruin your trip. I learned that, through bitter experience.

The first time I traveled to Europe, I had just separated from my first husband and didn't know where I was going. My first destination was the south of France, which meant bathing suits, black tie outfits and south-of-France-type beachwear. But I didn't know where I'd go after that. Maybe Paris, Rome, London . . . ?

Because I didn't know where I'd be going, I didn't know what I'd be needing. So I took everything. I had seven pieces of luggage and paid $345 (many years ago!) to get it on the plane.

I stayed in St. Tropez, and was shanghaied in the middle of the night by Harold and Grace Robbins. I ended up on their yacht, stayed on it for a week with enough luggage to travel around the world, slept in a stateroom with two valpaks, and the big joke of the entire south of France was Polly Bergen and *her luggage*.

It was torture, absolute torture. I just hated it, because I was a slave to my luggage. People may have been comfortable traveling that way in the days when they were pulled by horses and accompanied by valets, nannies and lady's maids. Nowadays it's ludicrous and a nightmare. If money is no object, break up your trip, come home and repack your luggage. But never do what I did that summer when I traveled like a snail with everything I had.

A European Tour

A dressy restaurant is dressy no matter where it is and a little informal place is always informal. Every woman should accept that what works for her in her home town will work anywhere in the world. It's only her own insecurity that makes her feel: When in Rome, do as the Romans do. If she tries, it won't work. Instead, when in Rome, do as you do in Des Moines or wherever you come from.

However, each place does have its own character, and it doesn't hurt to have a general idea of what that is. Just as you change slightly with each person you meet, and you'll sometimes even *consciously* adapt yourself to a new person, so you make little adaptations to the country or city you're in.

But this book isn't intended as a travel guide. The clothes you wear in London are the same as those you'd wear in New York, which are the same as those you'd wear in any cosmopolitan city. Since London is often the first stop for American tourists, and since many tourists will visit London no matter where else they go in Europe, London has its own section (earlier in this chapter). To have a section on each city in Europe would become monotonous—the differences aren't great enough.

So here are only a few notes on a few places, based on my own observation, that will hopefully be helpful hints:

Dressing for Rome

If you're going in the summer, be prepared to swelter. Rome gets extremely hot, much hotter than Paris, and you'll probably want to do all the walking you can before the heat overwhelms you. You'll wear sundresses, little tops, no stockings and open sandals. For Rome, the country-peasant look is right and the most comfortable.

Take only a couple of things for evening wear. Rome on the whole is not dressy—for a tourist. If you're visiting Italian friends, that may be another story. Italian women, like Spanish women, are often extremely elegant and go in for high-fashion designer clothes. The Italian woman is romantic, Latin, volatile. She likes romantic, flowing, exotic outfits, unlike the Parisian woman, who tends to be understated, to wear clothes with simple chic.

If you're staying in a hotel and don't foresee any big occasions, you won't need much evening wear in Rome. A long peasant skirt is romantic, feminine and airy—perfect for strolling past the Coliseum at twilight.

For Rome, as for all of Italy, as well as for Spain and Portugal, be

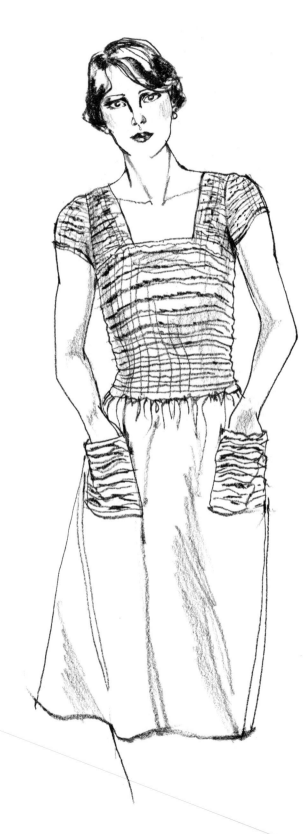

When in Rome...

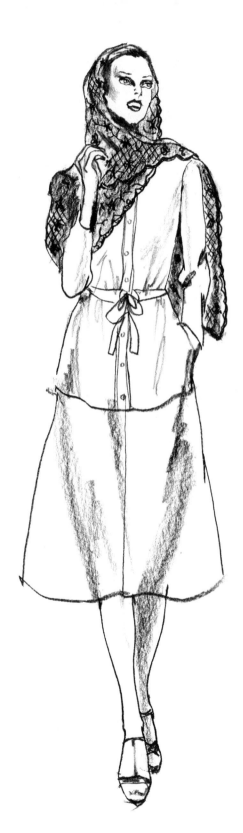

. . . be discreet.

sure to pack a large kerchief (in black lace if you have it) to wear when you enter churches. All countries that take their Catholicism seriously require that a woman's head be covered in church. If you're in Spain, get an exquisite mantilla, an old handmade one if you can find it.

In any city, a tight skirt is a bad idea, and particularly in Europe. Many old cities have a lot of steps leading up to monuments, cathedrals or city walls. In Greece, for example, you'll be climbing steps a lot of the time, as you will in Prague. Straight skirts will be uncomfortable, will tire you out and won't look attractive. Take loose skirts instead, with give to them, or straight-looking skirts with inverted pleats; or take culottes, that look like a skirt when you're standing still but give you complete freedom when you're walking or climbing.

Dressing for Vienna

Central Europe is slightly more formal than countries further west and provides more opportunities for opulence. The Viennese woman is less understated than the Parisian woman, but day wear is still quite casual. In Vienna, women dress in a slightly "prettier" or more "feminine" way than do women in other German-speaking cities, like Munich, Zurich or Frankfurt. (Munich is very close to Paris in terms of understated chic and elegant, simple cut in clothes.)

The opera house, Vienna's pride, was built for the Emperor Franz-Josef and his sumptuously beautiful empress, Elizabeth. Though the opening of the opera is a very dressy occasion everywhere, in Vienna it's particularly grand and glamorous, an opportunity to see men in tuxedos again. If you plan on going, take your most regal gown. You can wear it again to a command performance in England or at the Salzburg Festival.

When music comes to Salzburg in the summer, it brings kings and queens, dukes and princesses from all over the world. The large green stones around a woman's neck are actually emeralds, and the blue ring to match her eyes is an enormous sapphire. Here, to the strains of Mozart, Strauss, Verdi or Beethoven, old elegance returns. Men are in black tie or white tie; women's arms are sheathed in long gloves. If your ball gown has been waiting for decades to go out in public again, take it along to Austria in the summer.

Dressing for the South of France

After you've packed your bikinis and beachwear, take a few black tie outfits. A long, clinging column of black, white or whatever, unrolled from your suitcase (where you hardly noticed it) and dressed up with jewelry is perfect. Your sensational velvet pants suit will not get you in everywhere. If you're going to a casino anywhere in Europe, wear a long dress and be on the safe side. Many places will not allow you to enter in pants of any kind.

If you're at the Winter Palace in Monte Carlo, where a quarter of a million dollars is won and lost at a gambling table, or if you're dancing at New Jimmy's, Régine's, or dining at La Réserve or the Hôtel du Cap, your escort will be expected to be in a suit and tie.

You'll want to dress elegantly, even formally for these places, but don't bother to take along your showstoppers. A showstopper will work only one time—then it'll probably need dry cleaning and you'll have to lug it around with you wherever you go.

I advise *never* taking a showstopper when you travel. The only exception to this rule is if you're going to be presented to the Queen or the Pope.

Dressing for Madrid, Barcelona, Lisbon

Spanish and Portuguese cities are similar to Italian ones. They may be a teensy bit more conservative, but in all staunchly Catholic countries it's most tactful for you as a tourist to cover up just a little more than you ordinarily would. Always cover your head in a church, and if you have nothing to cover it with, don't go inside. Don't wear shorts or very short skirts—no minis. Don't call attention to youself by dressing in a way that will be considered brash. Even though you're a tourist, don't try to get away with clothes that would be considered improper on a Latin woman.

Remember that unchaperoned women are a new phenomenon in these countries and that until a few years ago, such women were considered either pros or easy marks. A tinge of that attitude remains, and if you're on your own, you'll probably be considered available. To get the message straight, and for your own comfort, go slightly more conservative in dress.

Dressing for Budapest to Moscow

Central Europe is a little more formal than France, and Eastern Europe is a little more conservative than Central Europe. In Poland, Hungary or Czechoslovakia, you'll see bikinis on the beach and women in long flowing beachwear. But when you go indoors—to a restaurant or a little theater—you'll find that the women have dressed up. In Paris, you can wear jeans to a theater or cabaret; in Prague, women are in what we'd call Sunday clothes.

Though beer parlors in East European countries invite casual dress (the traditional Western uniform of jeans is the most popular), a night out—to the opera, ballet, dancing—means evening clothes. Long dresses are not usually the free-flowing, easy gowns of the West. They have a more homey quality about them, as though made from brocaded upholstery material or drapes.

In Russia, you'll stand out as a Westerner no matter what you do. Don't try to dress down or in any way be patronizing in your appearance. Some Russian women are very well-dressed, and though fashionable garments are not so easily available there, women are interested in fashion and enjoy seeing what an American woman wears. Your super jeans pants suit is ideal for walking across Red Square. For the Bolshoi Ballet in the evening, wear one of your long noncrushables, with a shawl or jacket. Don't try for a very wealthy appearance, but don't go to the opposite extreme either. Casual elegance and good grooming are a pleasure everywhere.

Wherever you are in Europe, or anywhere abroad for that matter, don't take along any of your beloved scruffy garments. The oversized shirt with a frayed collar that you took over from your boyfriend may be your favorite thing to wear at home, and you may look great in it, but leave it at home, with all the other torn and faded lovables.

When you're traveling, you're clearly not in your own garden or kitchen. Your beat-up favorites will not seem interesting or eccentric on the streets of a European city or in village lanes. You'll simply look ungroomed and careless.

It's a mistake Americans sometimes make, particularly young Americans. It's tactless abroad, where people generally have less money to spend on clothes than we do, and where torn or scruffy clothes on a tourist (who had the money to get there, obviously) are seen as an affectation of poverty. Don't do it; whether you mean to or not, the message you give out will be insulting.

The same rule holds when you're in the countryside, particularly in the mountains. Inhabitants of mountainous countries take the mountains seriously. Don't go climbing in sneakers that are hanging on by a thread. If you're skiing, wear proper ski clothes. Worn-out jeans are not all right up in the Alps, where Alpinism is a way of life and ski teachers and mountain guides have gone through rigorous training to qualify for their positions. Often they are required to pass tests in a few languages. They take their jobs seriously, have learned first aid and are very careful never to expose a tourist to danger. If you come to the ski school in jeans with patches, you are showing disrespect for all the traditions of the country you're in. Avoid possible rudenesses by never packing anything that is in disrepair. Between casual and sloppy lies all the difference in the world.

Arranged Tours

For group tours anywhere, get in touch with the company or group leader and ask about clothing requirements. They'll tell you what weather, climate and occasions you should anticipate.

Outside Europe

South Americans, Asians and Africans all expect women to dress more conservatively or discreetly than Europeans or Americans do. In some countries, native women are still covered from head to toe and wear purdah. Be very careful not to offend. Unless you're familiar with the place and are absolutely sure it's okay, don't wear anything cut out. No bare midriffs or deep décolletés. Always cover up a little more than you think you should. Remember that in the hottest countries of all, natives often conceal the entire body.

If you're going on a safari, check with the company or group and they'll tell you what's needed.

In South America, where you would dress as conservatively as in Spain by day, you can let yourself go at night. South American night life is very swinging. You can wear the most décolleté, divine outfit you own, in the most exciting colors in the world. It's okay to bare it in Brasilia. And if you're in Rio during carnival time, anything goes (or comes off).

You're Going on a Cruise

Of all vacations, a cruise can be absolutely the most relaxing. You have no responsibilities, you're cradled by the sea, wherever you want to go is right there, and you don't even have to carry money. The sea voyage has always been recommended for health, and it's amazing to watch a stubborn flu that has resisted every kind of modern medicine, as well as old-fashioned bed-and-liquids therapy, suddenly shrink away to nothing on the high seas. The sea is the great restorer—of health, energy, spirits.

Whether you're on a passage or a cruise, in deluxe or tourist accommodations, this is a time out of time, when the world is far away, newspapers are forgotten and your life is buoyed up between the banks of past and future. It's a time to relax, unwind, no trouble about anything. It's also a time when you can be anyone you please. You don't ever have to see any of the passengers again, and nothing at all has to be serious.

Whether it's a weekend or a long cruise, whether you'll remain on board the whole time or disembark, it's best not to take much luggage. There's no penalty if you do, not in terms of money. There's no baggage allowance. If you're taking your pet elephant you won't be charged extra, as long as you can find a suitcase big enough to put it into.

While there's no penalty for a lot of weight, the problem is space. A stateroom is at best small, usually tiny. Even if you're in it alone, there's not much room, and if you take a lot of luggage, you'll find yourself sleeping with it. That isn't nearly as exciting as sleeping with somebody. Luggage, I've found, is not very responsive.

The less luggage, the freer you are. Also, there's not much hanging space (an important point to remember if the cruise is so awful that you want to kill yourself).

If the ship is making stops along the way, you'll need things to wear in port. A sundress and sandals, or other comfortable walking shoes, and a sun hat form a perfect outfit unless it's cool. In that case, a comfortable skirt or slacks and a top will do just as well. If you'll be staying till evening, take along a lightweight shawl. Put it in the large bag (straw?) you're carrying. You'll need the bag if you want to go shopping.

On shipboard itself, you'll need shorts, slacks, bathing suits, sundresses, skirts and tops. There will be at least one black tie evening, a gala night, so take an evening dress. It's more likely, on any extended cruise, that there will be at least two gala evenings a week (maybe more) so take along any evening dresses you want to wear.

You may, if you want to, wear a really grand dress, but a dressy caftan or a long jersey will do just as well. Because of the space problem, don't take more than one voluminous gown, and if that really takes up a lot of room, you'd do best to forget it. You'll wear it only once, and you might get sick of edging past it every morning when you go to brush your teeth.

If you're buying evening dresses for the cruise, select lightweight, long, simple ones—anything from highnecked to strapless style. You'll be able to take as many of these as you like—half a dozen won't take up the room of one ball gown. If you want to look really dressy, get them in dressy fabrics, or in brilliant colors. Or dress them up with jewelry, or tie diaphanous scarves around them for the layered look. Gold belts are sensational on long, lean dark dresses, but if you're overweight, substitute long gold chains for the belt.

On a cruise, your décolleté can take a plunge. The barer the better. You can go backless, strapless or with a V to the navel. If you're a librarian who has to wear "sensible" clothes every day, here's your chance to dress like a vamp. Let your fantasies and your body show. The woman in the slinky scarlet with large diamond cut-outs on the sides is probably a kindergarten teacher.

On almost every cruise, there's a costume night. Try to pack some things that you might be able to work into a costume, like large scarves or fringe numbers. I'd forgotten about costumes once when I was on a cruise, and I was very hard put to create something appropriate for Apache night. Common for costume nights are the Left Bank (French artist) or Buccaneer/pirate themes: the sea or "bohemian" motifs. A flesh-colored body suit is a great item to have. You can wrap scarves around it, sew things onto it or even paint on it. Any body suit is good, but a flesh-colored one is most exciting and adaptable to any costume.

A marvelous accessory to have for costume night or any night, on sea or on land, is a flower. Fresh flowers are beautiful, but hard to find in the middle of the Atlantic or even in your hotel room when you're getting ready to go out. So pack some of those lovely artificial flowers that you can roll almost to the size of a cigarette. When you take one out of your suitcase, push it open and flatten it out with your fingers and you've got a perfect gardenia, or rose or whatever, to use any number of ways. At lunch, put it on a sheath; tie it around your neck with a ribbon or band; pin it on an evening gown or tape it to your shoulder with transparent tape if you're wearing a strapless gown. Wear it behind your ear, in your hair or, in the most flirty way possible, between your breasts. It's a wonderful accessory. It looks real, and you can dab a few drops of perfume or cologne on it if you think people will be coming close enough to smell. It's especially effective on a ship: gazing out at the moon with a white rose in your hair, a fragile stole over your naked shoulders, you'll seem a vision from the romantic age.

Daytime on the cruise is for relaxing, swimming, tanning or sipping long cool drinks with a warm man at your side or a juicy book in your hands. Don't worry about your daytime clothes. Let them be comfortable and easy, and you'll feel that way too.

For evening, let yourself go in any direction you'd like: sleek and sophisticated, feminine and romantic, sultry, mysterious—whatever you'd like to be. Nighttime on shipboard is a chance to get all decked out.

An Island in the Sun

For the tropical island paradise, you take basically the same wardrobe you'd pack for a cruise, though you might have to leave out a few items if you're going by plane.

As with every trip, what you take depends largely on where you'll be staying and what you plan on doing. If you're renting a cottage for a week in the Virgin Islands with your husband or lover, you won't need more than one evening dress. Bright oversized scarves can work as long skirts or a long strapless dress as you sip your cuba libres on the balcony overlooking the setting sun.

But if you're staying at the Caribe Hilton, Dorado Beach, or any of the other large hotels in San Juan, you'll be in the casino or on the dance floor every night, and you'll need evening clothes for every evening you're there. They don't all have to be dresses; lounging pajamas and long skirts will allow you greater variety through mixing and matching. Pack things that are color-coordinated, so that three evening outfits will enable you to wear something different for ten nights. A long, easy skirt in a silk synthetic or lightweight knit can be worn with any number of tops, and the tops will go with the pants of your pajamas. If the pajama top is a jacket, you can make it into a three-piece outfit. Or wear the jacket over a long dress.

For all warm islands, pack the swimming and beachwear described in the previous chapter (see "In the Swim"). You'll need four bathing suits if you plan on swimming daily and don't like getting into a soggy suit. Many hot places are humid as well, and the suits won't dry out quickly. No matter where you're going, never pack only one bathing suit. Any time you need one, you need at least two. And if swimming will be your main activity, do take four. That frees you for a swim before breakfast, a morning on the beach or at the pool, an afternoon swim—and an extra suit for a midnight swim or for a change in case the wet bathing suit becomes uncomfortable. Anyone with even a touch of bladder problems should change out of a wet bathing suit immediately. And if you're menstruating, you'll probably want to.

Four bathing suits, a fun bathing cap, a beach wrap or cover-up, beach shoes or sandals, kerchiefs and a hat, sunglasses and lots of large scarves are all you'll need for day, unless you plan to go into the town. If you do, take a sundress or skirt along. Pants might get very hot and sticky, particularly over skin that's been sanded, salted and creamed. Shorts may or may not be appropriate, and you'll only know that after your first time out and a look around. But even if they're okay for shopping, they will definitely not be appropriate for lunch, and they will—or *should*—keep you out of any churches you might want to visit. If the island is Catholic, you'll need a covering for your head, as in Spain or Italy. But your head will probably be covered anyway; the salty air, sun and humidity rarely improve a coiffure.

Evening wear will be determined by where you are, and with whom. If your dress or top is bare, always take something for warmth. The hottest tropical island can get as cold as the desert at night.

No matter in what season you go, no matter how hot the weather you can expect, don't go anywhere without packing a jacket, sweater or stole. You'd be best off with all three. Not only are the nights generally cool, but there's always a chance of breezes and even strong winds coming along the ocean. Also there may be rain. Take your summer coat, the light-colored duster. It should be waterproof. If it's not, or only good enough for drizzle but not for tropical downpours, take a plastic raincoat. A trench coat looks fine, but will probably be too warm. A rain hat, bonnet or just a little plastic kerchief is essential. Take at least one extra plastic kerchief. Keep it in the pocket of your raincoat or inside your handbag. It takes up almost no room and is the most necessary of all emergency items to have handy in case of rain.

Almost any island you go to, from Majorca to Martinique, will require the same wardrobe. For French islands, you may only need your bathing suit bottoms on the beach, but take the tops along to wear with your large scarves.

If your tropical paradise is on the mainland, you may need a few town clothes. Wherever the place is not mainly built around tourism, most people will be leading a normal working life and your beachwear on the streets would be tasteless. If you're going to a Muslim country, you'll have to cover up even more than in a Catholic one. Though a bikini may be all right on a North African beach, you should dress in an old-fashioned ladylike way for the market place or the casbah. That doesn't mean gloves and stockings—a peasant skirt and blouse are fine. But don't wear something that insults the women and mocks the men.

In these countries, I would not wear my large scarves with a tiny top. I would cover myself up more. A djellaba, worn commonly by Muslim men, is a wonderful loose garment that covers you completely, but is wide enough to let the breezes come through and cool you off. It's generally white with dark gray or black stripes and has a hood to protect your head and hair.

People from temperate climates take off their clothes in the sun, but people in the tropics often cover themselves up as protection against the heat. The covered-up look can be very beautiful. Sheer white fabrics in a loose cut that don't bind the body are not only cool and crisp to the eye, they also make you feel cooler. Tanned arms and shoulders under a light, almost transparent, veil of fabric look wonderful and exciting.

If you're going with a group or on a package tour, don't be afraid of asking ahead of time what to pack. People are often ashamed to admit that they don't know what to take. But there's absolutely nothing wrong with calling up and asking the head of the group. It's what the Queen of England and her husband would do if they planned to tour a new country. The British ambassador to that nation would be called and asked what clothing requirements there are for their Majesties. He'd then give a rundown of places and occasions and appropriate dress.

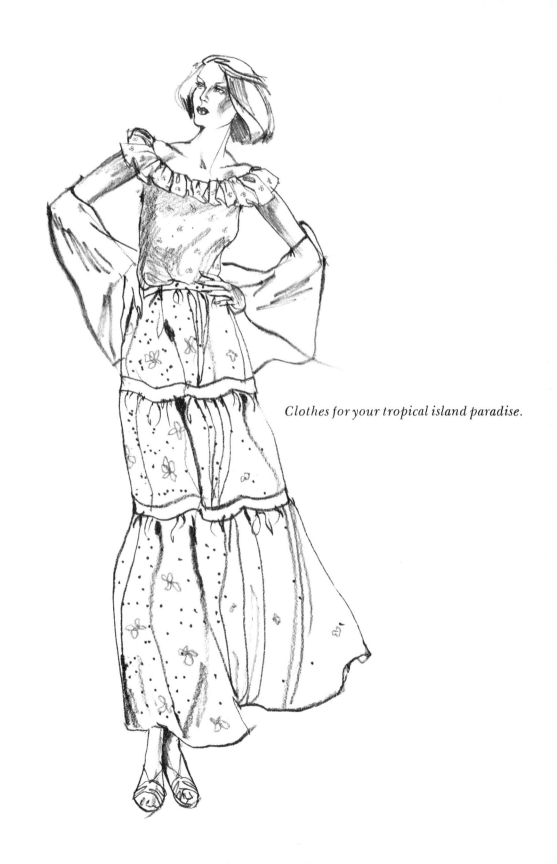

Clothes for your tropical island paradise.

Different groups set very different requirements. Club Med, for in-stance, is determinedly informal. Your spangled evening dress would never be worn on a Club Med vacation, even in the dressiest country. So it's always best to check ahead of time.

It's very important to know what weather you can expect whenever you're traveling. When I travel to any place in this country for busi-ness, I always call the weather report of that city ahead of time. For anywhere in the United States and Canada, dial the area code and WEather 6-1212. You'll get the weather report for that day, and a pre-diction for days ahead.

When you'll be traveling abroad, you can call the international weather bureau. Some newspapers (the *New York Times*, for instance), give you yesterday's weather in cities all over the world. But if you want to know in advance what weather and climate you can reason-ably expect in a country at a particular time of year, call the consulate or the information service.

Or rely on what the group leader or coordinator tells you. (Unless he confesses he's never been there before.) In any case, when in doubt, ask. There's absolutely no point feeling insecure about your wardrobe when one phone call can solve your problems. Don't think you'll be showing off your ignorance by asking and that everyone will know this is your first trip abroad. The most experienced travelers ask. Heads of state always ask. It's a necessary part of protocol.

A Note on Las Vegas

Instead of Nassau, you're splurging on Vegas. You've waited years to have one big blast. The money's saved up, no point in waiting any longer; you're taking a week off from work, both of you are, and you'll blow the whole bundle in fun and excitement.

From five o'clock in the afternoon on, you can wear the dressiest, most outrageous, most décolleté, most exciting clothes in the world. But maybe you'll be seated next to a lady who will have on blue jeans and a sweat shirt. Anything, absolutely anything, goes in Las Vegas. You can be as overdressed, underdressed or undressed as you want to be. You can take everything you own or just two pants suits, one for day and one for night. Wear one on the trip, pack the other and you'll have everything you need.

Or go the other route: Get the jewels from the family vault, wear gowns dripping with pearls; pour yourself into a Mae West hourglass strapless in black spangles and carry a boa. You will be overdressed, but what the hell.

For daytime, pack whatever you like wearing—shorts, skirts, pants or dresses. Take bathing suits if you plan to go swimming.

There are no rules, not even any faint guidelines for what to wear in Vegas. The only important thing to remember is the weather. In the summertime it's absolutely unbearable, it's so hot. You'll be most comfortable in the barest kind of clothing you own—while you're outside.

When you go inside, you freeze. Everything is extremely, overly air-conditioned; you have the sensation of walking from a furnace into a freezer. You positively need something to wear over your shoulders.

In the wintertime, Las Vegas is comfortable, but it's not hot. It's not like Florida. On two occasions in the last twenty-five years it has even snowed in Vegas. So realize you're not going to a hot resort in the winter. The climate will be more like spring or fall. But except for the jacket, there is absolutely nothing you should or shouldn't take. Las Vegas is like some mad opening at a modern art museum which is theoretically black tie, but where people come in everything from jeans to ball gowns, with everything in between and a few really incredible costumes.

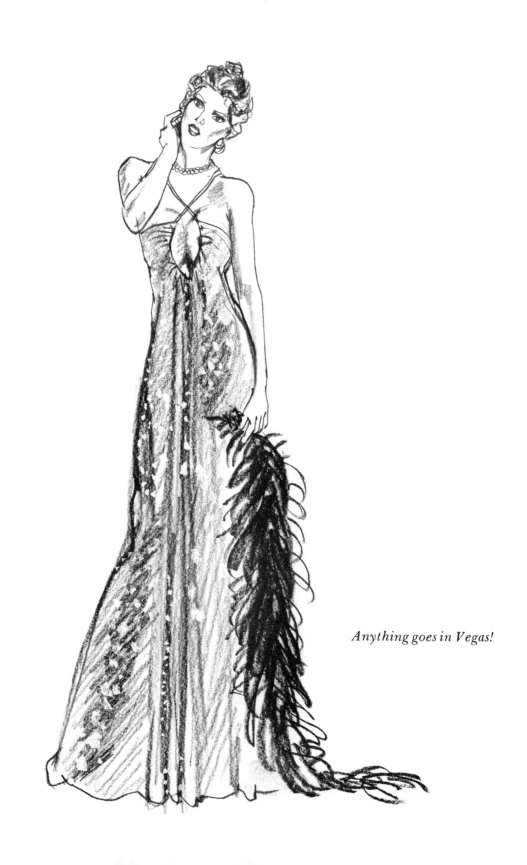

Anything goes in Vegas!

What's Right for Beauty Farms,
Health Spas, Nudist Camps

At a spa or beauty farm, you'll be spending most of the day in shorts, bathing suit, exercise outfit (yours or theirs) or naked. If the emphasis is on health, you won't have to bother much about your clothes. Dress will either be prescribed ahead of time in the brochure or instructions you're sent or you can assume it's informal. You'll need a couple of pairs of pants with blouses and sweaters, and one long skirt for a possible festive evening.

Most beauty farms are not co-ed. At Maine Chance, the Golden Door and others, you probably won't leave the premises during your stay. Going into the town disrupts your beauty day and disturbs your diet. So you'll remain at the farm, exercising, swimming, tanning, sweating in the sauna, being massaged, getting a facial, manicure, pedicure, getting starved and falling exhausted to sleep. You'll be with other women, most of whom are here primarily to lose weight. (Exceptionally few come to gain weight, and some come because of alcohol problems or just to escape.)

Evenings, you don't have to dress for your cranberry-cocktail hour or your melba toast dinner. Take along what you'd wear at home in the evenings, unless the brochure of your particular place specifies more formal dress. Maine Chance is more formal than the Golden Door, for instance—but you are told that in the printed information.

Take comfortable clothes for the climate and don't try to make a fashion statement. It will only come across as competitive in an atmosphere where women are working, individually and together, to lose weight and become more attractive.

Co-ed beauty farms and health spas can be more formal, even dressy—particularly European health spas. Don't try to predict what you'll need; *ask*.

Years ago the spa—or "watering place"—was among the most elegant places you could go. Spas meant not only health (they were usually built around mineral springs), but also gambling, dancing, entertainment and the full elegance of high society. The Romans considered baths so essential that no settlement was built without a bathhouse. Important business was transacted there, sumptuous meals were eaten, wine was drunk, and the whole thing led to Roman orgies.

In the eighteenth century the town of Bath, England's most elegant watering place, was also the hub of fashion. The master of ceremonies of the entire town (especially of the gaming tables) was Beau Nash, and he was given the name "Beau" because of the way he dressed. Women had special gowns made for going to Bath, which represented the height of competitiveness in dressing.

Now, even in Europe, people go to spas more for health than for fashion. Probably the best-known of all European health places is the Bircher-Benner clinic in Switzerland. It's known for its diets and cures, not for its games and clothes.

But there's absolutely no way to figure out the clothing requirements for any of these places. Some are self-contained, others are part of a town or city. Some have "seasons," like a resort. If you go to Saratoga Springs, for example, you may need clothes for the race track and the night life.

Health resorts are the most unpredictable places of all, since they range from totally informal to very dressy. For the actual health and beauty routines, you'll be in exercise or sweat suits wherever you are. But at night it's anyone's guess, and I strongly advise you don't try making your own.

A nudist camp is one place where you can avoid the necessity of making choices. Your birthday suit is fine for most occasions. If you feel it's grown a little worse for wear, you might try rouging nipples or knees, or even consider a paint job for the whole body. You might want to take your lashes, wig, your silicone implant or your merkin (pubic wig).

For evening wear, a ring might be appropriate, or a dab of perfume. Avoid overdressing! If you don't want to put on anything more than the TV, feel free.

Seriously, if you *do* go to a nudist camp, the best thing to leave behind is self-consciousness. I once went to one, out of curiosity, and at the beginning I was afraid to take my clothes off. I was sure everyone would be staring at me. Of course, what happened was that people stared because I was clothed.

It took me a while to realize that this was not a competitive situation. Most people, I think, are afraid to take off their clothes because they're sure everyone else has the body of a Miss or Mr. America. But that's not so. People who choose nudity because it makes them feel healthier are not interested in showing themselves off. When everyone is nude, I've found that nudity is no longer provocative.

Whatever is covered is more exciting than what's exposed. When women wore long skirts, the sight of a well-turned ankle drove men to rapture. Not many men will go wild over an ankle today. Where women are braless, either on beaches or in societies that have never required women to cover their breasts, breasts are not nearly as exciting as they are in places where they're never exposed in public.

When you're at a nudist camp or on a nudist beach you forget the fact that you're naked. You're responding to the sun and water on your body. If you want to be an exhibitionist, wear a bikini. Or cover everything in a high-necked, long-sleeved evening dress, with maybe just one slit at the side. Everyone will be staring at the slit.

Dressing for Business Trips and Conventions

The clothes you will need on business trips have been basically covered in the section on business, though they will depend on the kind of business you've come to do and where you're doing it. If you'll be touring factories, your clothes should naturally be more understated than if you're having a high-level meeting at the Watergate. Some of your business might include luncheons or evening meetings.

In all cases, a suit with silky shirt or blouse or a simply-cut dress— a sheath or shirtwaist—will be appropriate. In some instances, a nice pants suit will work, particularly in cool weather, but the jeans suit, no matter how well cut or how expensive, is definitely out.

Choose clothes that won't wrinkle or become otherwise disheveled-looking during a long workday. Put an extra pair of stockings or panty hose in your bag, in case of emergency. Other useful things to carry with you, in a bag or briefcase, include: makeup bag, comb and brush, atomizer, silk scarf, jewelry, delinter or small clothes brush, rain bonnet or kerchief, as well as the notebook, pens and appointment book you'll need for business.

If you'll be meeting people for the first time, particularly if they're not accustomed to dealing with women, it's very important to dress in a professional, businesslike manner and still not compete with the boys. Don't try to look mannish; though you want people to deal with you no differently than with a man, they'll find it a lot harder to do if you seem to be disguising your sex. You're a business person first in this situation, but you're also a woman—always. So don't play games in either direction. Walk the narrow path between obvious femininity (which gives a hint of helplessness, or at least nonserious-ness) and a mannish appearance, which gives the impression you're in disguise, that you've gotten yourself up to compete directly with the boys on their level.

If you're not sure how the evenings will go, it's better to be safe than embarrassed. You may be dining with other women—those who work in the office or the wives of men you're doing business with. If your clothes make a competitive statement, the evening becomes strained. Don't take along anything very bare unless you have a strong inkling you'll need it. Otherwise, let your evening clothes match the tenor of your day clothes: chic and understated. Take a long skirt, a long simple dress, a dinner dress or a reasonably covered-up cocktail dress. If you don't know whether you'll be going to restaurants or be invited to someone's home for dinner, the dinner dress is a perfect choice.

You won't want to take a lot of luggage with you for a short business trip. You may be going directly from the airport to a meeting. You probably won't be spending much time in your hotel room and you won't have the opportunity to make many changes. Leave your lounging clothes at home, along with your jeans and showstoppers, your fun clothes, your outrageous outfit and your strapless sheath. To be completely safe, don't take your peasant clothes along either. Stick to the simplest lines you have.

For a trip of only a few days, you won't need more than the suit you have on, another suit or dress with jacket for daytime, a couple of long skirts or a long dress and a simple dinner dress. Take a change of tops and accessories that will go with the different outfits, to dress them up or soften them.

For a convention, you won't go wrong if you follow the same suggestions, particularly if you add a cocktail dress. But there are conventions and then there are conventions. Some are held in resort hotels, where you'll have a chance to swim or play tennis. Evening clothes at this kind of place will probably be quite dressy. You might be going to cocktail parties in public rooms or in the privacy of someone's suite.

What kind of a convention are you headed for, and are you participating directly or accompanying your husband? If it's the kind of convention where spouses come along, you can dress up more than if the convention is limited to participants. You'll have time to dress and so will the other women. This is a vacation for you, even if it's business for him, and a chance for a woman to wear clothes she likes but rarely has an opportunity to wear at home.

If it's strictly business, whatever the business, there will still be a few prearranged social events and you will undoubtedly know about them before you go. If a barbecue has been planned, take a peasant skirt or pants. For a seated dinner reception, take a short or long evening dress.

If it's your first convention, don't rush out and buy special clothes. Let's say you're a librarian going to the American Library Association convention. You'll see a few people you know, and you might meet the man of your dreams. It's a break in the routine, you're determined to make the most of it, and whatever else happens, you'll have fun.

Great. Just don't assume that the others have invested two months' salary in a new wardrobe. You know what clothes your colleagues generally wear to work, and you can safely assume that those are the same ones they'll take along to the convention. You have some idea who will be there and what their general life-style is. Do they wear pants or gowns in the evening? If the convention is for librarians, don't dress up in clothes people might wear at a stockbrokers' convention.

Ask yourself the following questions before you pack for that business trip or convention:

Where you'll be staying. The more expensive the accommodations, the dressier the clothes. Daytime chic, and evening formal.

Are wives and girlfriends invited? If so, even if you'll be taking part in the meetings all day, remember that the other women will have the time and inclination to dress up. Don't try to be competitive, but you can afford to be feminine at night. If no escorts or spouses are coming along, the convention is serious business and you probably won't need anything formal.

What events have been planned? You'll be sent a list of scheduled meetings and social events before you leave. Take clothes appropriate for the specified occasions.

What is the nature of the business? Academic conventions will be more casual than business conventions. If heads of large corporations are convening, there's a greater possibility of a black tie dinner than at a convention of biochemists.

In what part of the country will you be, and at what type of hotel? If the convention is in Sea Island, Georgia, you'll naturally need resort clothes. Take them along for conventions at any of the large resort hotels in the Catskills, too. At Grossinger's or the Concord, and similar places, you'll have a choice of sports and other shipboard-type activities during the day. At night, clubs will offer dancing and entertainment.

If the convention is in a large city or industrial town, you need city clothes. If the evening is not planned, you'll choose your own form of entertainment and, depending on who you are, will either need pants for bumming around, a suit for the theater or an evening outfit for a nightclub.

Remember that most people at the convention will be much like you in life-style and style of dressing. They or their husbands do the same work you do or your husband does. Don't think a convention is like Cinderella's ball. If it's a convention of Cinderellas, everyone will be in rags; but if it's a convention of Prince Charmings, everyone will be in the usual old ball gown and glass slippers.

One-day Trips

For the day trip that includes spending the night somewhere, you'll need some luggage. But take only what you can comfortably carry yourself. When I take the shuttle flight from New York to Washington on business, I always carry my luggage on and off the plane to save time. I've developed unbelievable muscles doing it, but I'm in a hurry and can't afford to stand around waiting for my baggage to come up from the hold.

I generally take a hanging bag and a duffel bag. The hanging bag is a one-suiter, in which I put the cocktail or evening dress I plan to wear that night and maybe a suit for the following day. In the duffel bag I carry all little items and my makeup and cosmetics. I always pack a steam blower, because I find I never seem to get to a hotel until after the valet service is closed and I'm off in the morning before it opens. So the steam blower is an essential. You plug it in, it blows out steam and you have an instant press before you go out at night or before you get dressed for your morning meeting.

If you won't be staying overnight, you obviously don't take luggage. You just have to be extra sure to choose clothes that will wear well throughout the day.

Perhaps you live in a suburb and plan to spend the day in the city. You take the train or car in the morning. You'll be shopping, going to a museum, having lunch with a friend, perhaps meeting someone for dinner and the theater later. You dress as though for a business day leading directly into evening. That means the knit suit or dress, with accessories in your bag and a makeup bag for touching up in the evening. You'll want to make sure your shoes are really comfortable so you won't have to change your plans because of aching feet. Your bag—a shoulder bag gives the most freedom—should be large but not heavy. You'll want room for small purchases and the newspaper or magazine you'll read on the train.

If you wear something on your head, a kerchief or turban is fine, but a large hat will get in the way. You'll never need gloves unless the weather is cold and you're wearing them exclusively for warmth. Don't try to protect your hands from dirt by wearing gloves. It's always easier to wash your hands than to send your gloves out for dry cleaning or even to wash them yourself.

Particularly if you plan on walking most of the time, support hose will be an extra comfort and can help prevent fatigue. Since you'll be carrying extra hose anyway, you can slip into the ladies' room and change into a sheerer pair in the evening. That's also the time to add jewelry. If you love dangling earrings or bracelets, wait till evening to put them on. They're really not suitable for daytime and will be disconcerting even to you as their jingle and clang accompany you throughout the day.

If your evening will be quite dressy, you won't want to deck yourself out at 8:00 A.M. in clothes that won't be appropriate for another ten hours. Remember: Underdressing is always better than overdressing. You may not be able to find the clothes that are the perfect compromise between morning shopping and the evening party, but a well-tailored black suit is an excellent beginning. Wear a shirt or blouse with it by day. In the ladies' room, before your evening appointment, you take off the blouse (a synthetic that you can roll up into your handbag) and put on the little halter top you've brought along. Or just leave off the blouse and wear the suit by itself with jewelry. There is almost nowhere, except a ball, where you won't be appropriately dressed. Just make sure you have a delinter or clothes brush along to freshen up the suit.

If the evening won't be formal or if it's open-ended, your best bet is to wear a skirt. There is no place that will not let you in if you're wearing a skirt—but there still are some places that may refuse you entrance in pants.

And even if you're going into the city to buy the suit or dress you'll want to wear in the evening, take the precaution of wearing something

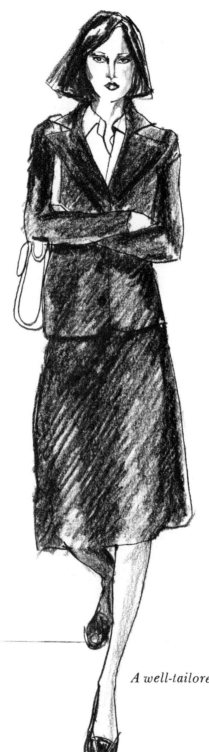

A well-tailored black suit is perfect for day . . .

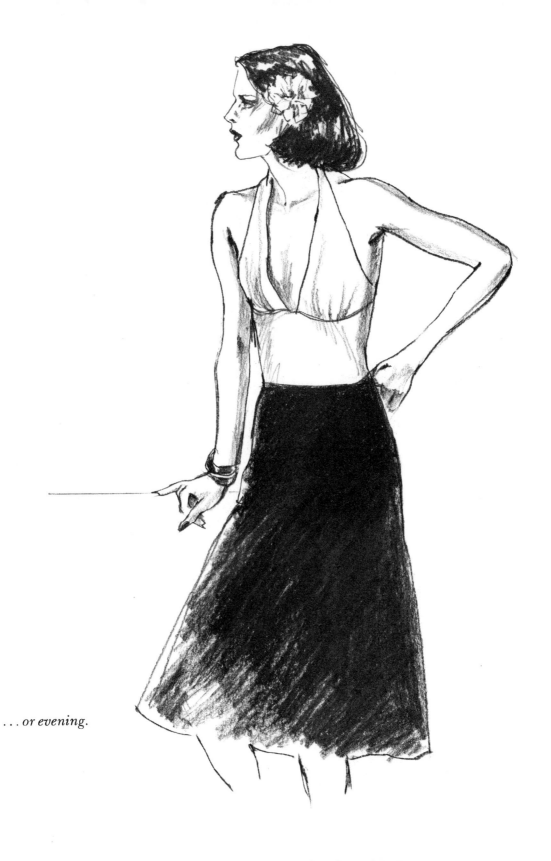

. . . or evening.

that will work, just in case you don't find what you're looking for and end up with nothing, or with a gorgeous see-through lace nightgown you picked up on sale.

Getting There

They say that getting there is half the fun, but it can also be a bore, particularly if you're riding in the car all day. Even beautiful scenery and a pleasant travel companion won't stop the fidgets. After a long day's drive, you should be rewarded with a nice dinner. So you want to be as comfortable as you can all day and still look good in the restaurant.

I find I'm usually more comfortable in a skirt than in pants. Pants can get too hot. Their other drawback is that those you're most comfortable in while riding won't look good when you stop. And if you wear well-fitting pants in the car, it's agony. They fit well, so they're tight and bind you when you're sitting in them all day.

Of course there are those marvelous pants that feel as good as they look. They're rarely jeans, though. And even if they are, the jeans that give you the greatest comfort while traveling won't get you into the places where you might want to go when you stop.

I have a pair of pants that do work and I wore them on my last long car trip. They're lightweight gabardine in navy blue. I wore a navy blouse, a V-necked sweater that went over the blouse, and a cardigan—in reds, blues and beiges—that matched the V-neck. I started off at 7:30 in the morning, rode in a car, continued on by plane, went to a meeting, stopped in a very nice restaurant for dinner and arrived home at 3:00 in the morning. I'd traveled for nearly twenty hours and didn't really look much the worse for wear. At 3:00 A.M. I still looked pretty much as I had when I'd set out at 7:30 the day before.

I wore the pants and blouse in the car, pulling on the sweater when

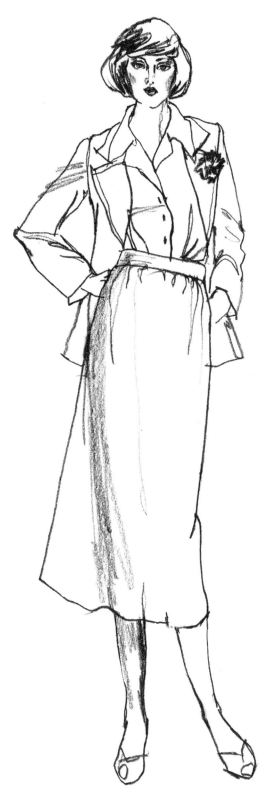

Be comfortable in the car and look good when you get there.

I felt cool. At the restaurant, I went to the ladies' room, brushed and delinted the outfit, put on the jacket and a silk scarf—and I was ready for the nicest restaurant anywhere.

A pants suit is great if it has enough give to be comfortable and resist wrinkles, while at the same time being chic. If you have such pants, they're perfect for cool weather. In warm weather, stick with skirts.

When a car trip is really long and you'll be stopping overnight, don't forget to pack a special valise for the motel. After a long, hard day you don't want to lug ten pieces of baggage just because one contains shoes, the other night clothes, another toiletries and so forth. Pack what you'll need for the night and the following day in a separate bag, and don't let that bag be the first piece of luggage you put in the trunk. When you travel, you don't need extra work or a Marx Brothers circus scene.

The World Cruise in the Greatest Possible Luxury

The best accommodations on the *Queen Elizabeth 2* will cost you $125,000 for the 1977 cruise around the world in eighty-one days. If you're embarking in Port Everglades, Florida, and not in New York, the fare will be $200 less, and you'll be cruising for only seventy-seven days.

This is an ideal jaunt for Texas oil millionaires, though if you're on a limited budget, you can get passage for as low as $6,950. You'll have to share your little inside room and toilet. You'll need some extra spending money for tips, drinks, laundry and all the expenses associated with your shore excursions, including port taxes and transportation to and from the ship. But still, if you watch your pennies, you should be able to do the whole thing for $10,000.

It'll be a frugal world cruise, though. You won't have room for much luggage, so you'll probably have to leave most of your furs and ball gowns at home. If you take the suite instead, you can comfortably bring along the four wardrobe trunks that accompany some passengers onto the *Queen Elizabeth 2*. For complete luxury and comfort, buy an additional stateroom, adjoining yours, for all your bags and baggage. This was done on the *France* when she toured the world. The stateroom that was engaged only for luggage was by no means luxurious—it merely cost $10,000.

For those who want to return to days and nights of splendor, this is probably as close as the modern world will let them come. But even here, white tie and tails are never required. To wear that sumptuous attire, go to the opening of the Vienna opera house.

Old-style ornateness is dying very quickly, as the air age replaces all other forms of transportation. No longer does June mean farewell champagne parties on board the *Andrea Doria*, the *Nieuw Amsterdam* or the *United States*, guests spilling out into the halls and stewards rushing with vases for all the flowers brought to the stateroom. No longer does November mean a leisurely cruise on Moore-McCormack Lines down past the Equator, stopping in Brazil, on to the tip of Argentina and then up past Chile and Peru, with dancing till dawn, casinos, floor shows, children's parties and riotous nights for adults.

Now, if you want to travel in grandeur, you're more or less stuck with Cunard's last great luxury liner. It makes twenty-four stops between leaving New York in mid-January and returning in early April. You'll be in most ports for only one day, though you have two in Rio de Janeiro, Brazil; two in Capetown, South Africa; two in Bombay, India; two in Bali, Indonesia; four and a half in Hong Kong; two each in Yokohama, Japan, and in Honolulu.

Don't take all eighty of your ball gowns. Even here, you won't have the chance to wear half of them. While you're in port, there are no galas, nor is there one the night before you arrive nor the night when you leave a port. Sadly, for those with the wardrobe of an empress and no chance to wear it, you will have only twenty-three grand possibilities for your stupendous gold filigree with pearls, your velvet with ermine and heavy brocade set with tiny diamonds around the neckline. So don't bring more than twenty-three imperial outfits—you really won't be able to wear more.

And don't bother packing *all* your furs, either. For most of the cruise the weather will be warm or even hot. Your sable will be fine for embarking in New York in January. If you're lucky, it will be one of those years when Florida has a cold spell and you can still be furred two days later. But then you can forget about it until you arrive in Los Angeles near the end of March—and not even the best contacts with the U.S. Weather Service could insure that you'll be in weather cool enough to wear your chinchilla. By the time you return to New York, it's April. It *may* be snowing, but still there's really very little point in taking more than three fur coats.

Even your fur stoles won't be able to come up for air too often. You'll definitely want to take your black Russian broadtail stole, of course, and your ermine just in case, but leave the others home in storage.

Do take *all* your jewelry, or as much of it as you can fit in one good-size wardrobe trunk. Having all that choice will allow you to spend many hours every day deciding which to wear.

To guarantee many leisurely hours of clothes-planning while on board, take all your summer clothes, two dozen bathing suits, fifty scarves, ten pairs of sandals and four dozen other pairs of shoes. Take all your handbags except the obviously wintery ones. Fifty sundresses will give you plenty to choose from. Take the same number of tops, but only twenty skirts—more than that is simply excessive.

You'll need shorts and pants, cocktail dresses, many negligees and lounging outfits (for private parties in your suite). You'll need dinner dresses for the nights before and after reaching port. Since you expect to be dining at the captain's table, you'll surely not want to wear the same dress more than once.

On any normal shipboard day, you can easily accomplish six changes of clothing. (Anything more than that will require a bit of ingenuity.)

After breakfast in bed in your satin café au lait peignoir over your lace negligee, you will change into pool clothes. Bathing suit and cover-up or wraparound are all you need, with a pretty sun hat, designer sunglasses and custom-made sandals. You will not have to change for shuffleboard, ping pong or the 11:00 A.M. bouillon in your deck chair.

Before lunch, you return to your cabin to put on a pretty little crisp dress of white sharkskin, with a soft red belt, red shoes and simple jewelry of gold or platinum. You go for drinks and, yes, you'll wear the same outfit straight to lunch. After lunch, you take everything off and give yourself a little beauty rest in the altogether or in a lightweight robe. When you rise, you put on your afternoon outfit, depending on what you plan to do today. For more swimming, you'll wear another bathing suit with a different cover-up. For a workout in the gym, you'll wear shorts and top or a leotard. For the movies or board games, take one of your light-colored pants suits with a silk blouse.

When evening comes, it will be time for your daily visit to the beauty salon and masseuse. You will not have to change. Only when you return from these appointments do you have to start preparing for evening.

For greatest effect, it's best to wear a cocktail dress or simple dinner dress for cocktails and dining, then return to your stateroom after dinner to get yourself into the grand gala, those hundreds of layers of thinnest silk wafting you gently toward the ballroom, diamonds sparkling in your ears, discreetly matched by a few more tiny diamonds scattered through your hair.

After the ball is over, you'll sink gratefully into bed in your simple, clinging gown of silk washed with the colors of the sea. In the morning, you call for your breakfast and reach for your matching peignoir.

On days in port, your opportunites to change will be severely limited. You and all your fellow oil millionaires will spend your day in the Seychelles or in Ceylon looking much like any other tourist in a $400 sundress or designer pants.

If you have the required time, the money and no responsibilities to keep you at home, you shouldn't be sitting there reading this book. Get on the phone now, make your reservation for the world cruise—and start packing.

7

The Importance of Clothes

As I've tried to convey all along, clothes are a very important form of nonverbal communication. They immediately reveal many things about you: your position in society, your age, your background, economic level, and many other things.

There are certain signals (like wearing clothes intended for the opposite sex) that everyone in our society agrees about. The woman who wears men's clothes and has very short hair will be regarded in the same way by almost everyone. And most of us would form the same first impressions of a woman wearing a poured-into outfit or of a man in a thin pin-striped suit. The woman is intent on one thing only and so is the man, though they're obviously on different trips: The woman is out for pleasure, the man for business.

Other signals given by the way we dress are read differently depending on who's getting the message. A straight, simple Halston on a Beautiful Person will be interpreted as the height of chic by some, and as too plain or unglamorous, by others. A turquoise outfit with matching hat, earrings, shoes and bag will strike the executive woman as dated and provincial; but the wearer of this outfit and her husband and friends will think she's pretty as can be in her Sunday-go-to-meeting clothes.

Your clothes will be making a statement on different levels. First, the overall statement that almost everyone interprets the same way: Are you male or female? Do you like the opposite sex or your own? Then: Are you rich or poor? (Though the range between the two extremes will be seen differently depending on where the observer stands.) Are you going out for work or for play? Are you a mature woman or still a girl at heart? Secure or insecure? Almost everyone from the same society will agree on the answers.

Then you will be appraised by your peers. They'll notice aspects of your dressing that others won't. At a rock concert, even a simple dress may mark you as stuffy and belonging to an "antique" generation while at a symphony concert, jeans would indicate disrespect.

You're judged differently by insiders and outsiders. A good example of this is at a gallery opening. Artists, friends and patrons form an "inside" group and dress for each other. They'll sometimes wear outfits that seem outrageous to outsiders, but the inside group interprets them as fun or imaginative. At an Andy Warhol–Jamie Wyeth opening in New York, attended by celebrity guests in the arts, a Queens truck driver commented to a *New York Times* reporter: "It's nice to see the rich people come out. But no matter how much money they have, they don't know how to dress right. Look at that blonde. Plastic shoes, no bra, too much makeup. Ridiculous! It's just not the right thing to wear to an art gallery."

"The right thing"—everyone has his own notion of what that is, even today, when dressing is freer than it ever was. Unspoken rules are still followed. You notice an immediate change in the people around you if you go from sloppy jeans and oversize shirt to a well-tailored suit. When you're projecting "class," you'll get better service from everyone and your word will be trusted more.

If you're in an expensive department store wearing designer clothes and you attempt to leave with an unpaid-for purchase in your hand, you'll be gently reminded that you made a mistake; could you please return this item? If the situation is the same except that you're wearing unkempt clothes or give a slovenly appearance, the reminder in all likelihood will not be gentle at all and you'll have a lot of explaining to do.

Behind what seems to be total freedom, there's still an unshakable code. Though it's adapted to the times (such as the acceptance of pants for women in places where they weren't accepted five years ago), the basic rules remain. Everyone can crack them.

When a person wonders what to wear, he or she is already limited to certain possibilities. Everyone in this society has been programmed to a certain extent and if the question is "What'll I wear to the dinner party?", we already know that the answer won't be a grass skirt, a mechanic's uniform or a tennis dress. Everyone is imprinted with at least a broad outline of what is appropriate where. We don't put on ski clothes to go to bed or wear black tie to a picnic.

"What'll I wear?" actually means: "Given this occasion, what can I put on that's appropriate and also looks good on me?" The less experience you have with a certain occasion, the less you'll know what to wear. A housewife who goes marketing regularly won't have a problem deciding what to put on for the supermarket—but she'll probably seek advice if she's been invited to the White House for the first time. The First Lady will instinctively know what to wear to a luncheon, but will consult with others on what to take for her trip to China.

What you have in your closet reveals your life-style. If you spend your days riding a tractor, your wardrobe will certainly be very different from the businesswoman's. If your social life means poker, bridge or the movies, you won't have (and won't need) the evening gowns of a woman who's often invited to dine and dance.

Every society wears clothes of some kind, and they always mean more than just protection or modesty. Some one from another culture might not be able to interpret the meaning of various types of clothes, but is sure to recognize that some kind of rules are being followed.

A Trobriand Islander might not be able to tell what's conveyed by a pin-striped suit as against khaki pants with matching sports jacket, but every American knows that a different message is being sent. Even though we're often not conscious of it, we respond to the language of clothes.

To a Martian, all earth people might seem to be using the same language. To a Chinese, all Westerners dress alike. But a Frenchman can spot an American in Paris by his clothes. A midwesterner knows a New Yorker when he sees one. A New Yorker can tell if you're from Flatbush or Park Avenue. In each case, the distinctions leap out at the beholder.

Though we can often tell what part of the country a person comes from by his way of speaking, we recognize that he's speaking English, and that it's specifically American English. The same goes for the language of clothes—just about everyone in America gets the same message (consciously or unconsciously) from certain ways of dressing.

Generally:

Jeans: "I'm young, casual, no-fuss, natural."
Business suit: "I'm in charge, I know what I'm doing."
Frills, ruffles, dirndls and pinafores: "I'm just an old-fashioned girl, romantic and dependent." They can also mean: "Poor little me is helpless and needs big strong you for protection."
Sportswear: "Thanks anyway, but I'll do it myself" or, "Let's do it together."
Simple lines, expensive fabric: "I'm top echelon/high society." They basically mean chic.
Out-of-date clothes: "I don't care, I can't be bothered."
Soiled, torn clothes: "I don't give a damn. I don't care what you think of me, because I don't think much of myself."
Doll-like dressing: "I don't know who I am."

Though you can never *completely* determine what message will be received by any particular individual, you can be sure you're saying a lot about yourself in the way you dress. You're saying who you are, or who you think you are, or who you want others to think you are.

Beyond that, you're also using clothes to conceal defects of your body, to change your mood, to project different aspects of yourself. Clothes will let you play games and enter into fantasy. Dressing is an art, a language and a game all people play. How well you play it will determine how clear your statement is. Your goal should be to play the game well enough so that your appearance always says. "This is me, this is who I choose to be."

By whatever means you're traveling, except possibly by balloon, you'll need clothes to keep you warm and keep you cool, by sun and candlelight, with princes or paupers. Here's a basic checklist, flexible enough to be adapted to your particular plans and style.

Around the World in 80 Items

Bras	3
(flesh color goes with everything)	
panty hose or stockings (with garter belt)	10
panties	10
(let at least one pair be very frilly or sexy)	
pants—casual (including jeans)	2
pants—dressy (evening)	2
shirts	3
sweaters/cardigans	6
(can also be sweater sets)	
other tops (jerseys, tunics, halters, etc.)	5
suits (with skirt or pants)	2

jackets	2
(one of these should be outerwear—fur, leather, heavy wool)	
raincoat/duster	1
winter coat (fur?)	1
stole (evening)	1
long dresses	3
(flowing: caftans, long T's; one of these can be lounging pj's; or take only one long dress and two long skirts)	
day dresses (these can be simple dinner dresses also)	3
scarves (in all or any sizes)	8
shoes (dark or leg-colored)	2
shoes for walking, exercise	1
(boots, sneakers, rubber soles)	
sandals	1
evening slippers	1
bed slippers	1
robe/peignoir	1
nightgowns	3
handbags	2
(black or earth colors)	
evening bag	1
(gold or silver)	
skirts	3
(long or short, depending on whether your suits have skirts or pants)	
grand gala, super-sensational	1
outrageous something-or-other	1
Grand Total:	80

For those of us who "have nothing to wear," here is the solution:

The Magic Three-piece Suit

Jacket and Pants

1. alone, with jewelry or scarf (ascot)
2. with blouse, shirt or top in same color
3. with silk man-tailored shirt
4. with shirt or sweater and scarf (ascot) tied at neck or worn into neckline
5. numbers 2, 3 and 4, alone, with a vest.
6. with a bright overblouse or tunic
7. a vest with jewelry or scarf.

Repeat 1-7 for jacket and skirt = 17
Repeat 2-7 for pants alone = 21
Repeat 2-7 for skirt alone = 25

Multiply the variations almost infinitely through belts or scarves at the waist or, with an overblouse or sweater, at the hips. Jewelry will stretch possibilities even further. Headwear, handbags, stockings and shoes can match or contrast with any outfit.

Choose jacket, skirt and pants in a nonseasonal, no-wrinkle fabric and in a neutral or dark color which can then be set off by tops and accessories. With these, you could go for weeks or even months without ever wearing the same thing twice. What top you choose will dress it up or down, and jewelry or other accessories can change the outfit from casual to dressy within seconds. If you don't wear a bra, don't forget the possibilities in unbuttoning!